MILAD
STANDARD COSMETOLOGY

EXAM
REVIEW

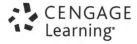

CENGAGE
Learning·

Australia • Brazil • Japan • Korea • Mexico • Singapore • Spain • United Kingdom • United States

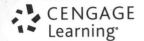

Milady Standard Cosmetology Exam Review, 2016 Edition

Author(s):
  Milady

Executive Director, Milady:
  Sandra Bruce

Product Director:
  Corina Santoro

Product Manager:
  Philip I. Mandl

Senior Content Developer:
  Jessica Mahoney

Associate Content Developer:
  Sarah Prediletto

Product Assistants:
  Harry Garrott
  Michelle Whitehead

Senior Director of
  Sales and Marketing:
  Gerard McAvey

Marketing Manager:
  Elizabeth Bushey

Senior Production Director:
  Wendy Troeger

Production Director:
  Patty Stephan

Senior Content Project
  Manager:
  Nina Tucciarelli

Senior Art Director:
  Benj Gleeksman

Cover image(s):
  Hair by Ted Gibson.

Photography by
  Joseph and Yuki Paradiso

Makeup artist:
  Valenté Frazier

For product information and technology assistance, contact us at
Cengage Learning Customer & Sales Support, 1-800-354-9706

For permission to use material from this text or product,
submit all requests online at **www.cengage.com/permissions.**
Further permissions questions can be e-mailed to
permissionrequest@cengage.com

Library of Congress Control Number: 2 0 1 4 9 5 0 2 7 9

ISBN: 978-1-2857-6955-4

Milady
20 Channel Center Street
Boston, MA 02210
USA

Cengage Learning is a leading provider of customized learning solutions with office locations around the globe, including Singapore, the United Kingdom, Australia, Mexico, Brazil, and Japan. Locate your local office at: **international.cengage.com/region**

Cengage Learning products are represented in Canada by Nelson Education, Ltd.

For your lifelong learning solutions, visit **www.milady.com**

Purchase any of our products at your local college store or at our preferred online store **www.cengagebrain.com**

Visit our corporate website at **cengage.com.**

Notice to the Reader

Publisher does not warrant or guarantee any of the products described herein or perform any independent analysis in connection with any of the product information contained herein. Publisher does not assume, and expressly disclaims, any obligation to obtain and include information other than that provided to it by the manufacturer. The reader is expressly warned to consider and adopt all safety precautions that might be indicated by the activities described herein and to avoid all potential hazards. By following the instructions contained herein, the reader willingly assumes all risks in connection with such instructions. The publisher makes no representations or warranties of any kind, including but not limited to, the warranties of fitness for particular purpose or merchantability, nor are any such representations implied with respect to the material set forth herein, and the publisher takes no responsibility with respect to such material. The publisher shall not be liable for any special, consequential, or exemplary damages resulting, in whole or part, from the readers' use of, or reliance upon, this material.

Printed in the United States of America
Print Number: 01 Print Year: 2015

CONTENTS

PREFACE

This book of exam reviews contains questions similar to those that may be found on state licensing exams for cosmetology. It employs multiple-choice questions, which have been widely adopted and approved by the majority of state licensing boards.

Groups of questions have been arranged following each chapter of the *Milady Standard Cosmetology* textbook. To get the maximum advantage when using this book, it is advisable that the review of subject matter take place shortly after its classroom presentation. After completing the chapter exams, use the answer key located in the back of the exam review to confirm the correct response. For this edition, the page number also appears of where to locate the answer in your 2016 edition of *Milady Standard Cosmetology*.

This review book attempts to keep pace with and ensure a basic understanding of infection control, anatomy, physiology, and salon business applicable to the professional cosmetologist. It also covers important topics such as client consultation guidelines, chemical safety in the salon, and basic procedures as well as some of the more advanced and creative aspects of the profession.

While the exam review serves as an excellent guide for the student in preparing for their state licensing examination, it is can also be beneficial for the experienced cosmetologist. It provides a reliable standard against which professionals can measure their knowledge, understanding, and abilities.

Furthermore, reviewing this material will help students and professionals alike to gain a more thorough understanding of the full scope of their work as they answer questions regarding practical cosmetology performance skills and related theory. Because the reviews are written for the most recent edition of the *Milady Standard Cosmetology* textbook, use of this material by professionals also helps to ensure that they have the most recent knowledge and information available to them in the industry.

CHAPTER 1 HISTORY & CAREER OPPORTUNITIES

1. African civilization had a variety of hairstyles that were used as a symbol of tribal traditions and conveyed a message of age, marital status, _____, and rank.
   a. political position
   b. religious beliefs
   c. power
   d. education ____

2. Which of the following civilizations was the first to infuse essential oils from the leaves, bark, and blossoms of plants for use as perfumes and for purification purposes?
   a. Chinese
   b. Egyptians
   c. Romans
   d. Greeks ____

3. The ancient _____ were the first to cultivate beauty in an extravagant fashion.
   a. Egyptians
   b. Romans
   c. Greeks
   d. Chinese ____

4. To achieve a look of greater intelligence during the Renaissance, women _____.
   a. wore highly colored lip preparations
   b. dyed their hair black or dark brown
   c. wore plain, simple clothing
   d. shaved their eyebrows and hairline ____

5. During the Middle Ages, women wore colored makeup on their _____.
   a. ears
   b. hands
   c. lips
   d. eyes ____

6. In ancient Rome, hair color was used by women to indicate _____.
   a. personal wealth
   b. class in society
   c. marital status
   d. education level ____

7. The ancient Greeks made lavish use of perfumes and cosmetics for grooming, medicinal purpose, and _____.
   a. religious rites
   b. burial rites
   c. social rites
   d. family events ____

8. During the _____, women commonly used henna to stain their hair and nails a rich, warm red.
   a. Egyptian Era
   c. Renaissance
   b. Victorian Age
   d. Middle Ages _____

9. If you were a middle-class woman in ancient Rome, you would color your hair _____ to indicate your class status.
   a. brown
   c. blond
   b. black
   d. red _____

10. Victorian women _____ to induce natural color.
    a. applied rouge
    b. pinched their cheeks
    c. applied lip stains
    d. applied natural ingredients _____

11. The onset of _____ led to a new prosperity in the United States, during which all forms of beauty began to follow the trends set by celebrities and society figures.
    a. World War I
    c. industrialization
    b. the Great Depression
    d. assembly lines _____

12. The makeup developed by _____ was popular with movie stars because it would not cake or crack, even under hot studio lights.
    a. Max Factor
    c. Mary Kay
    b. Charles Revson
    d. Charles Nessler _____

13. Gloria Swanson and _____ helped glamorize the hip new nail lacquer trend in the 1930s by wearing matching polish on their fingers and toes.
    a. Marilyn Monroe
    c. Elizabeth Taylor
    b. Lillian Gish
    d. Jean Harlow _____

14. By 1925, the Associated Master Barbers and Beauticians of America (AMBBA) established the National Education Council with the goal of standardizing requirements for barber schools and barber instructor training, establishing curriculum, and setting forth _____.
    a. shop protocols
    b. service prices
    c. state licensing laws
    d. a professional dress code _____

15. The world's first ammonia-free haircolor was invented by
_____ in 1985.
- **a.** Vidal Sasson
- **b.** Farouk Shami
- **c.** Trevor Sorbie
- **d.** Noel DeCaprio

_____

16. _____ holds the key to individual development
and personal motivation, gives you knowledge and
confidence, and provides you the best opportunity to
advance your career and achieve real success.
- **a.** Continuing education
- **b.** Networking
- **c.** Basic school education
- **d.** A professional attitude

_____

17. A _____ provides a connection between salons
and their staff and the rest of the beauty industry by
providing information about new products, new trends,
and new techniques.
- **a.** salon trainer
- **b.** manufacturer educator
- **c.** haircolor specialist
- **d.** distributor sales consultant

_____

18. In order to get experience providing hairstyling services on
film and TV sets, you should be prepared to _____
for a period of time.
- **a.** work only a few hours a day
- **b.** offer to volunteer
- **c.** work without implements
- **d.** immediately join a union

_____

19. To be a successful salon manager, you must have an
aptitude for math and accounting and understand
_____.
- **a.** anatomy
- **b.** marketing
- **c.** chemistry
- **d.** physiology

_____

20. The curling iron was invented by _____.
- **a.** Vidal Sassoon
- **b.** Max Factor
- **c.** Marcel Grateau
- **d.** Sarah Breedlove

_____

21. Most manufacturers consider the creative director to be
_____ and the driving force behind brand success.
- **a.** an executive-level position
- **b.** a mid-level position
- **c.** a low-level position
- **d.** a first-tier position

_____

22. In 1932, Lawrence Gelb, a New York chemist, introduced the first permanent haircolor product and founded a company called _____.
- **a.** L'Oreal
- **b.** Nexus
- **c.** Wella
- **d.** Clairol

_____

23. The individual credited with coining the term *day spa* is _____.
- **a.** Sarah Breedlove
- **b.** Marcel Grateau
- **c.** Noel DeCaprio
- **d.** Madam C.J. Walker

_____

24. The beauty icon who turned the hairstyling world on its ear with revolutionary geometric cuts was _____.
- **a.** Max Factor
- **b.** Vidal Sassoon
- **c.** Charles Nessler
- **d.** Queen Nefertiti

_____

25. The second half of the twentieth century saw the introduction of tube mascara, improved hair care and nail products, and the boom and _____ of the weekly salon appointment.
- **a.** death
- **b.** proliferation
- **c.** growth
- **d.** wane

_____

2 LIFE SKILLS

1. Short-term goals are those goals that can generally be completed within one _____ or less.
   a. day
   b. year
   c. month
   d. week ____

2. Which of these terms refers to the moral principles by which we live and work?
   a. Equality
   b. Emotions
   c. Ethics
   d. Justice ____

3. The ability to deal with difficult circumstances comes from having _____.
   a. well developed life skills
   b. specific career goals
   c. a fine-tuned smile
   d. a strong family unit ____

4. All of the following are reasons why cosmetologists should study and have a thorough understanding of life skills *except:* _____.
   a. having good life skills eliminates the need for self-esteem
   b. well developed life skills will help you deal with difficult circumstances
   c. practicing good life skills leads to a more satisfying and productive career
   d. life skills help you keep interactions with clients positive ____

5. Which of the following is one of the Action Steps for Success?
   a. Always strive to meet your salon manager's definition of success.
   b. Show respect only for those people who can help you in your career.
   c. Never practice new behaviors.
   d. Keep your personal life separate from your work. ____

6. Which of the following is one of the recommended strategies for effectively managing your time?
   a. Make effective time management a habit.
   b. Do not schedule free time into your day because free time is a waste of time.
   c. Always work as hard as possible, even if it means neglecting physical activity.
   d. Plan your commitments around your leisure time. ____

7. Effective communication is improved through practicing nonverbal and verbal skills, as well as _____.
- **a.** having a warm smile
- **b.** active listening
- **c.** talking softly
- **d.** speaking loudly ____

8. In order to be diplomatic, you should be assertive rather than _____.
- **a.** aggressive
- **b.** intelligent
- **c.** sensitive
- **d.** considerate ____

9. It is recommended that you study during blocks of time that would otherwise be wasted, such as while _____.
- **a.** getting sufficient rest
- **b.** practicing new skills
- **c.** listening to your instructor
- **d.** waiting in a doctor's office ____

10. When we pay attention to our _____, we can learn how to manage our time efficiently.
- **a.** insecurities
- **b.** cravings
- **c.** inner organizer
- **d.** feelings of guilt ____

11. Self-esteem is based on inner strength and begins with trusting your ability to _____.
- **a.** communicate with others
- **b.** achieve set goals
- **c.** become popular
- **d.** handle clients effectively ____

12. An unhealthy compulsion to do things perfectly is called _____.
- **a.** punctuality
- **b.** procrastination
- **c.** professionalism
- **d.** perfectionism ____

13. The conscious act of planning your life, instead of just letting things happen is described as having _____.
- **a.** ambition
- **b.** a game plan
- **c.** goals
- **d.** dreams ____

14. _____ or negative thoughts can be counterproductive and work against your ability to succeed.
- **a.** Unsure behavior
- **b.** Vigorous exercise
- **c.** Self-critical
- **d.** Frequent naps ____

15. Putting off until tomorrow what you can do today is called _____.
- **a.** time management
- **b.** procrastination
- **c.** perfectionism
- **d.** scheduling ____

16. To achieve success, it is important to make a conscious effort to _____ everyone.
    a. respect **c.** admire
    b. criticize **d.** believe in ____

17. Three bad habits that can keep you from maintaining peak performance include not having a game plan, seeking perfectionism, and _____.
    a. failing to prioritize **c.** procrastinating
    b. annual planning **d.** making mistakes ____

18. One Action Step for Success suggests that you practice doing whatever helps you maintain _____.
    a. an elevated ego
    b. a positive self-image
    c. a comfortable demeanor
    d. a friendly approach ____

19. Procrastination may be a symptom of _____.
    a. lacking a game plan
    b. taking on too much at one time
    c. a compulsion for perfection
    d. exceptional organization ____

20. _____ involves fulfilling one's full potential.
    a. Self-indulgence **c.** Self-management
    b. Personal desire **d.** Self-actualization ____

21. Which of the following blocks the creative mind from exploring ideas and discovering solutions to challenges?
    a. Criticism **c.** Familial support
    b. Motivation **d.** Enthusiasm ____

22. How long should your personal mission statement be?
    a. A brief summary **c.** One or two sentences
    b. One or two paragraphs **d.** One or two pages ____

23. When setting feasible goals, it is important to _____.
    a. lock into a rigid plan
    b. create a plan and revisit it often
    c. avoid frequent changes to the plan
    d. focus on what feels good today ____

24. When you ensure your behavior and actions are aligned with your values, you maintain your _____.

    a. self-image   **c.** motivation

    b. ethics   **d.** integrity   ____

25. Motivation and self-_____ skills will help you move to the next level in your career.

    a. esteem   **c.** involvement

    b. centeredness   **d.** management   ____

3 YOUR PROFESSIONAL IMAGE

1. While working, your clothing should always be stylish, comfortable, and _____.
   - **a.** highly accessorized
   - **b.** formal
   - **c.** functional
   - **d.** colorful ____

2. Your _____ involves your posture and the way you walk and move.
   - **a.** physical fitness
   - **b.** physical presentation
   - **c.** physical problems
   - **d.** physical activity ____

3. The way to counter the negative impact of repetitive motions or long periods spent in one position is by _____.
   - **a.** stretching and walking around at intervals
   - **b.** wearing ill-fitting shoes
   - **c.** practicing regular body manipulation
   - **d.** being aware of the body vascular system ____

4. There are consequences to not maintaining a professional image in the salon including loss of clients, a poor reputation, and _____.
   - **a.** loss of self-esteem
   - **b.** a bad attitude
   - **c.** having fewer friends
   - **d.** loss of income ____

5. Your shoulders should be relaxed and _____ when you are providing client services.
   - **a.** slightly curved
   - **b.** level
   - **c.** slightly arched
   - **d.** extended ____

6. One weak moment of _____ right before performing a service because you did not plan ahead could spell disaster.
   - **a.** drinking coffee
   - **b.** texting a friend
   - **c.** posting on Facebook
   - **d.** calling a friend ____

7. The science of designing the workplace as well as its equipment and tools to make specific body movements more comfortable, efficient, and safe is _____.
   - **a.** economics
   - **b.** ergonology
   - **c.** ergonomics
   - **d.** ecology ____

8. The daily maintenance of cleanliness by practicing good healthful habits is _____.
   a. personal hygiene
   b. physical presentation
   c. professional image
   d. professional hygiene _____

9. The impression you project through both your outward appearance and your conduct in the workplace is _____.
   a. personal hygiene
   b. physical presentation
   c. professional image
   d. professional hygiene _____

10. Which of these items should be kept in your hygiene pack?
    a. Lipstick
    b. Toothbrush
    c. Teeth whitener
    d. Gum _____

11. As a professional cosmetologist, you should brush and floss your teeth and use _____ throughout the day as needed.
    a. lotion
    b. antiseptic
    c. fragrance
    d. mouthwash _____

12. In addition to being free of dirt, it is important that your clothing is _____.
    a. stain free
    b. new
    c. expensive
    d. colorful _____

13. To help protect your clothing from dirt and stains, consider investing in _____ to wear at work.
    a. a pair of scrubs
    b. an apron or smock
    c. a pair of coveralls
    d. scotch-guarded clothing _____

14. Ensure you are dressed for success by tuning in to _____.
    a. your innermost desires
    b. the weather and environment
    c. the salon's culture
    d. your career goals _____

15. Your shoes should have a low heel and _____.
    a. offer good arch support
    b. have a tight fit
    c. have a soft sole
    d. have a loose fit _____

16. As you work, your neck should be _____.
   a. bent over the client
   b. elongated and balanced above the shoulders
   c. leaning toward the dominant hand
   d. leaning away from the dominant hand   ____

17. One goal of ergonomics is to make workplace tools safer and more _____.
   a. attractive   **c.** economical
   b. flexible   **d.** efficient   ____

18. Negative gossip and _____ can bring an ideal atmosphere to a halt.
   a. poor listening   **c.** friendliness
   b. impolite demeanor   **d.** consideration   ____

19. An awareness of your posture and _____, coupled with good work habits, proper tools, and equipment, will enhance your health and comfort.
   a. height   **c.** movements
   b. weight   **d.** activity   ____

20. As you work, you should hold your elbows at no more than a _____-degree angle away from your body for extended periods of time.
   a. 60   **c.** 15
   b. 90   **d.** 25   ____

21. As you work, your wrists should be kept in a _____ as much as possible.
   a. straight or neutral position
   b. turned upward position
   c. bent position
   d. turned downward position   ____

22. As you work, a good guideline to follow is to _____.
   a. endure long periods of uninterrupted repetitive motions
   b. keep your back and neck relaxed
   c. avoid regular stretching exercises
   d. use ergonomically designed implements   ____

23. Repetitive motions have a cumulative effect on the muscles and _____.

a. bones

c. tendons

b. joints

d. skin

____

24. To avoid ergonomic-related injuries, consider using _____.

a. a back brace

c. an anti-fatigue mat

b. knee braces

d. a heated body wrap

____

25. Establishing a professional online image is an essential _____ attribute.

a. spiritual

c. personal

b. image-building

d. popularity-building

____

CHAPTER 4 COMMUNICATING FOR SUCCESS

1. Good communication skills reduce potential workplace
   _____.
   a. harmony
   b. compatibility
   c. conflict
   d. consistency
   ____

2. In handling a client who is dissatisfied with a service, the ultimate goal is to _____.
   a. convince the client that you are right and she is wrong
   b. make the client happy and willing to return for future services
   c. get the client out of the salon as quickly as possible
   d. fully satisfy the client, regardless of the cost
   ____

3. Effective human relations and communication skills build _____, accelerate professional growth, and promote a positive work environment.
   a. strong values
   b. professional ethics
   c. stimulating conversations
   d. lasting client relationships
   ____

4. The sixth step of the 10-Step Consultation Method is
   _____.
   a. review the intake form
   b. determine and rate the client's preferences
   c. show and tell
   d. discuss upkeep and maintenance
   ____

5. A practical step for effectively communicating in the workplace is to _____.
   a. be inattentive
   b. believe in yourself
   c. talk more and listen less
   d. react instead of responding
   ____

6. The ability to understand people is _____ to operating effectively in many industries.
   a. the key
   b. irrelevant
   c. incidental
   d. unimportant
   ____

7. To earn a client's _____ and loyalty, be consistent by always having a positive attitude.
   a. money
   c. trust
   b. affection
   d. respect _____

8. If a client requests a specific cut or color that she has seen on a celebrity that cannot be achieved, you should _____.
   a. create your own design ignoring what the client has specified that she would like
   b. refuse the service and tell the client this cut or color would not work for her
   c. perform the service since this is what the client has requested
   d. create a plan, offer alternative looks, and set future goals _____

9. You may want to schedule clients who are _____ late for the last appointment of the day or ask them to arrive earlier than their actual appointment time.
   a. habitually
   c. rarely
   b. never
   d. occasionally _____

10. When you meet an older client for the first time, you should _____.
   a. address the client by the honorific
   b. address the client solemnly
   c. address the client by their first name
   d. ask how the client wishes to be addressed _____

11. When interacting and communicating with coworkers, make every effort to remain _____ and resist being pulled into spats and cliques.
   a. assertive
   c. objective
   b. aggressive
   d. aloof _____

12. As a cosmetologist, do not attempt to fulfill the role of _____, career guide, parental sounding board, or motivational coach for any of your clients.
   a. haircolor expert
   b. counselor
   c. professional acquaintance
   d. polite listener _____

13. If a client is revealing increasingly personal details, one recommended strategy is that you _____ or find a reason to excuse yourself, and when you return, change the subject or suggest a mini relaxation service.
    a. change the subject
    b. reveal a personal detail
    c. discontinue the service
    d. turn on a loud machine _____

14. As you interact and communicate with coworkers, you should be honest and _____.
    a. oblivious   c. frightened
    b. sensitive   d. averse _____

15. When communicating with your salon manager about an issue or problem, it is recommended that you _____ beforehand.
    a. cover up your mistakes
    b. think of possible excuses
    c. think of possible solutions
    d. think of who you can blame _____

16. The act of successfully sharing information between two people (or groups of people) so that the information is understood is called _____.
    a. direct communication
    b. effective communication
    c. strong communication
    d. overt communication _____

17. The document also known as a client questionnaire, consultation card, or health history form is the client _____.
    a. intake form   c. greeting form
    b. welcome form   d. entrance form _____

18. The _____ is the communication with a client that determines the client's needs and how to achieve the desired results.
    a. client conversation   c. client consultation
    b. client communion   d. client conference _____

19. When should the client consultation be performed?
   a. Before starting the actual service
   b. During the service
   c. After the service
   d. When booking the appointment   ____

20. It is recommended that you allow how much time in your schedule to do the client consultation?
   a. 3–5 minutes   **c.** 1–3 minutes
   b. 5–15 minutes   **d.** 15–20 minutes   ____

21. The third step of the 10-Step Consultation Method is to _____.
   a. perform a needs assessment
   b. analyze the client's hair
   c. determine and rate the client's preferences
   d. review the client's lifestyle   ____

22. Your reactions to situations beyond your control and your ability to _____ in the face of challenges are critical to being successful in a people profession.
   a. stand up   **c.** control fear
   b. communicate effectively   **d.** remain assertive   ____

23. If you are involved with a scheduling mix-up, always remember to _____.
   a. be polite while arguing that you are correct
   b. be polite and never argue about who is correct
   c. be assertive and argue that you are correct
   d. be aggressive, but refrain from arguing   ____

24. One important golden rule of communication for building a successful beauty industry career is to _____.
   a. be aware of your body language
   b. speak softly
   c. use casual grammar and slang
   d. be casual and comfortable   ____

25. The ninth step of the 10-Step Consultation Method is to _____.
   a. review the consultation
   b. discuss upkeep and maintenance
   c. make color recommendations
   d. review the client's lifestyle   ____

CHAPTER 5 INFECTION CONTROL: PRINCIPLES & PRACTICES

1. Cocci are bacteria that are _____.
   a. round-shaped
   b. rod-shaped
   c. corkscrew-shaped
   d. spore-shaped
   ____

2. Which type of bacteria can cause strep throat or blood poisoning?
   a. Diplococci
   b. Spirilla
   c. Bacilli
   d. Streptococci
   ____

3. Bacteria that grow in pairs and can cause pneumonia are _____.
   a. diplococci
   b. bacilli
   c. staphylococci
   d. streptococci
   ____

4. Lyme disease and syphilis are caused by spiral or corkscrew-shaped bacteria called _____.
   a. diplococci
   b. bacilli
   c. spirilla
   d. cocci
   ____

5. A chemical process that destroys most, but not necessarily all, harmful organisms on environmental surfaces is _____.
   a. disinfecting
   b. sanitizing
   c. cleaning
   d. sterilizing
   ____

6. Bacteria generally consist of an outer cell wall containing a liquid called _____.
   a. nucleic acid
   b. cytoplasm
   c. protoplasm
   d. protons
   ____

7. The process whereby bacteria grow to their largest size, and then divide into two new cells is _____.
   a. binary fission
   b. meiosis
   c. photosynthesis
   d. metamorphosis
   ____

8. The presence of pus can be a sign of _____.
   a. immunity
   b. congestion
   c. a bacterial infection
   d. a sunburn
   ____

9. A _____ infection appears as a lesion containing pus and is confined to a particular part of the body.
   a. systemic
   b. local
   c. primary
   d. secondary
   ____

10. Which of the following is a condition caused by an infestation of head lice?
    a. Hepatitis
    b. Scabies
    c. Pediculosis capitis
    d. Tinea pedis
    ____

11. The ability of the body to destroy, resist, and recognize infection is called _____.
    a. immunity
    b. decontamination
    c. inflammation
    d. regulation
    ____

12. Disinfectants sold and used in the United States must carry _____ registration number.
    a. a Food and Drug Administration (FDA)
    b. an Occupation Protection Agency (OPA)
    c. a U.S. Department of Labor (DOL)
    d. an Environmental Protection Agency (EPA)
    ____

13. Which agency publishes the guidelines known as Standard Precautions?
    a. FDA
    b. OSHA
    c. CDC
    d. EPA
    ____

14. In 2012, OSHA agreed to comply with the Globally Harmonized System of Classification and Labeling of Chemicals System (GHS), which requires the use of a standard format called _____ (SDS) to replace the MSDS.
    a. Safety Data Support
    b. Surety Data Support
    c. Safety Data Sheet
    d. Safety Data Standards
    ____

15. A type of disinfectant with a very high pH that can damage the skin or eyes is called _____.
    a. alcohol and bleach
    b. EPA-registered disinfectants
    c. alcohol and quats
    d. phenolic disinfectants
    ____

16. When washing your hands, after you have used warm water, applied soap, and then rubbed your hands together until a lather forms, use a disinfected nail brush to brush your nails horizontally back and forth under the free edges and then up and down along the nail folds of the fingernails. The process for brushing both hands should take about _____.

    a. 5 minutes
    c. 45 seconds
    b. 60 seconds
    d. 10 seconds
    ____

17. Antiseptics are intended for _____.
    a. disinfecting instruments
    b. reducing microbes on the skin
    c. disinfecting equipment
    d. sterilizing equipment
    ____

18. Standard Precautions require employers and employees to assume that all human blood and body fluids are potentially _____.

    a. infectious
    c. dangerous
    b. harmless
    d. toxic
    ____

19. The SDS contains _____ categories of information.
    a. 10
    c. 14
    b. 12
    d. 16
    ____

20. When disinfecting a whirlpool foot spa after use by a client, you must circulate the disinfectant for _____ or the length of time indicated on the product label.
    a. 5 minutes
    c. 60 seconds
    b. 10 minutes
    d. 20 minutes
    ____

21. After cleaning and disinfecting a pipeless foot spa after each client, how should you dry it?
    a. With a clean paper towel
    c. With a blowdryer
    b. With a clean linen towel
    d. Let it air dry
    ____

22. Which form of hepatitis is the most difficult to kill on a surface?
    a. Hepatitis A
    c. Hepatitis C
    b. Hepatitis B
    d. Hepatitis D
    ____

23. Accelerated hydrogen peroxide (AHP) is a recently approved form of disinfectant that only needs to be changed every
_____.

    a. 5 days   **c.** 7 days
    b. 30 days   **d.** 14 days   ____

24. It is important to wear gloves and _____ while disinfecting nonelectrical tools and implements.
    a. remove jewelry   **c.** an apron
    b. safety glasses   **d.** a face mask   ____

25. Licensing, enforcement, and your conduct when you are working in the salon are regulated by _____ agencies.
    a. federal   **c.** city
    b. state   **d.** international   ____

26. Some _____ disinfectants are harmful to salon tools and equipment.
    a. antifungal   **c.** hospital
    b. nonporous   **d.** tuberculocidal   ____

27. As part of the SDS categories, first-aid measures include important symptoms/effects as well as _____.
    a. product use
    b. required treatment
    c. use restrictions
    d. containment and clean-up   ____

28. Cutting living skin is allowed only by _____.
    a. advanced nail technicians
    b. medical nail technicians
    c. qualified medical professionals
    d. advanced cosmetologists   ____

29. Fungal infections are much more common on the _____ than on the hands.
    a. face   **c.** elbows
    b. feet   **d.** knees   ____

30. Items that can be cleaned, disinfected, and used on more than one person even if the item is accidentally exposed to blood or body fluid are called _____.
    a. single-use   **c.** disposable
    b. porous   **d.** multiuse   ____

31. The process that destroys all microbial life is
_____.
   a. sanitization
   b. cleaning
   c. decontamination
   d. sterilization
   ____

32. If the label on a disinfection product includes the word *concentrate*, it means that the product must be
_____.
   a. used without water
   b. heated during use
   c. diluted before use
   d. heated before use
   ____

33. Quat solutions are _____ disinfectants when used properly in the salon.
   a. very effective
   b. somewhat effective
   c. never effective
   d. somewhat adequate
   ____

34. Using _____ bleach can damage metal and plastic.
   a. too little
   b. diluted
   c. any amount of
   d. too much
   ____

35. 5.25 percent sodium hypochlorite is also known as
_____.
   a. white vinegar
   b. household bleach
   c. household ammonia
   d. table salt
   ____

36. Never let disinfectants such as phenols come in contact with your _____.
   a. implements
   b. skin
   c. gloves
   d. clothing
   ____

37. Items that are _____ are also considered absorbent.
   a. phenolic
   b. parasitic
   c. pathogenic
   d. porous
   ____

38. It is recommended that salons identify each time a piece of equipment is used, cleaned, disinfected, tested, and maintained _____.
   a. in the cosmetologist's memory
   b. a note pad
   c. in a logbook
   d. in a private computer file
   ____

39. There is no additive, powder, or tablet that eliminates the need for you to _____ equipment.
    a. clean and sterilize   **c.** clean and maintain
    b. clean and disinfect   **d.** clean and immunize   ____

40. Not having _____ available poses a health risk to anyone exposed to hazardous materials and violates federal and state regulations.
    a. SDSs   **c.** HRVs
    b. MRSAs   **d.** CDCs   ____

41. Antimicrobial and antibacterial soaps are _____ regular soaps or detergents.
    a. slightly more effective than
    b. no more effective than
    c. just as effective as
    d. slightly less effective than   ____

42. _____ include guidelines for the use of gloves, masks, and eyewear when contact with blood or body secretions containing blood or blood elements is a possibility.
    a. Standard Preconditions   **c.** Standard Precautions
    b. Universal Provisions   **d.** Universal Preparations   ____

43. After they have been properly cleaned and disinfected, implements should be stored in a _____ container.
    a. permanently sealed   **c.** clean, uncovered
    b. disposable   **d.** clean, covered   ____

44. After each client, you should properly clean the basic foot basin or tub, and then add the appropriate amount of disinfectant and let it soak for _____ or the time recommended by the manufacturer.
    a. 10 minutes   **c.** 1 minute
    b. 5 minutes   **d.** 10 seconds   ____

45. Before beginning any service, you should wash your hands using pump soap, warm water, and a _____.
    a. chemical disinfectant
    b. clean, disinfected nail brush
    c. clean, disinfected sponge
    d. chemical exfoliant   ____

46. A disease that is spread from one person to another is called a(n) _____.
   a. systemic disease
   b. contagious disease
   c. toxin
   d. fungicidal ____

47. The one-celled microorganisms having both plant and animal characteristics are called _____.
   a. flagella
   b. fungi
   c. cocci
   d. bacteria ____

48. The transmission of blood or body fluids through touching, kissing, coughing, sneezing, or talking is known as _____ transmission.
   a. indirect
   b. infection
   c. sterile
   d. direct ____

49. Transmission of blood or body fluids through contact with an intermediate contaminated object such as a razor, extractor, nipper, or an environmental surface is known as _____.
   a. direct transmission
   b. direct portability
   c. indirect transmission
   d. indirect transference ____

50. Various poisonous substances produced by some microorganisms are called _____.
   a. tinea
   b. toxins
   c. bacteria
   d. flagella ____

51. A disease that is spread from one person to another person is _____.
   a. a communicable disease
   b. an infectious disease
   c. an occupational disease
   d. a systemic disease ____

52. A disease caused by pathogenic organisms that enter the body, and which may or may not be spread from one person to another person, is _____.
   a. a systemic disease
   b. an infectious disease
   c. an occupational disease
   d. a contagious disease ____

53. As part of the SDS 16 categories, toxicology information includes routes of exposure, related symptoms, and

    _____.
    a. safe handling and storage
    b. acute and chronic effects
    c. exposure and protection
    d. restrictions and transportation   ____

54. Any organism of microscopic to submicroscopic size is a

    _____.
    a. staphylococci   c. mycobacterium
    b. streptococci   d. microorganism   ____

55. The removal of blood or other potentially infectious materials on an item's surface, and the removal of visible debris or residue is called _____.
    a. disinfection   c. decontamination
    b. cleaning   d. sterilization   ____

56. _____ disease affects the body as a whole, often due to under- or over-functioning internal glands or organs.
    a. A systemic   c. An occupational
    b. An infectious   d. A contagious   ____

57. The determination of the nature of a disease from its symptoms and/or diagnostic tests is _____.
    a. an analysis   c. a direct transmission
    b. a disinfection   d. a diagnosis   ____

58. _____ is a condition in which the body reacts to injury, irritation, or infection.
    a. An allergy   c. A contagion
    b. An inflammation   d. An exposure incident   ____

59. A parasitic disease may be caused by _____.
    a. bacteria   c. lice
    b. bacilli   d. cocci   ____

60. A _____ is a submicroscopic particle that infects and resides in cells of biological organisms and is capable of replication only through taking over the host cell's reproductive function.
    a. cocci   c. bacterium
    b. virus   d. parasite   ____

61. The virus that causes AIDS is _____.
   a. hepatitis B virus (HBV)
   b. human papilloma virus (HPV)
   c. hepatitis C virus (HCV)
   d. human immunodeficiency virus (HIV)   ____

62. Contact with non-intact skin, blood, body fluid, or other potentially infectious materials that are the result of the performance of an employee's duties is _____.
   a. an allergy   c. a contamination
   b. an inflammation   d. an exposure incident   ____

63. The scientific name for barbers itch is _____.
   a. tinea capitis   c. folliculitis barbae
   b. tinea pedis   d. tinea spirilla   ____

64. Organisms that grow, feed, and shelter on or in another organism while contributing nothing to the survival of that organism are _____.
   a. cocci   c. parasites
   b. bacilli   d. debris   ____

65. The presence, or the reasonably anticipated presence, of blood or other potentially infectious materials on an item's surface or visible debris or residues is called a(n) _____.
   a. infection   c. inflammation
   b. contamination   d. allergy   ____

66. The term _____ describes a ringworm fungus of the foot.
   a. tinea capitis   c. tinea barbae
   b. tinea spirilla   d. tinea pedis   ____

67. A reaction due to extreme sensitivity to certain foods, chemicals, or other normally harmless substances is a(n) _____.
   a. allergy   c. inflammation
   b. contamination   d. infection   ____

68. _____ is produced by organisms, including bacteria, viruses, fungi, and parasites.
   a. A systemic disease   c. A pathogenic disease
   b. An infectious disease   d. A contagious disease   ____

69. Illnesses resulting from conditions associated with employment are _____.

    a. contagious diseases   **c.** pathogenic diseases

    b. occupational diseases   **d.** systemic diseases   ____

70. As part of the SDS 16 categories, handling and storage lists precautions for safe handling and storage, including _____.

    a. incompatibilities   **c.** reactions

    b. ingredients   **d.** identifiers   ____

71. The methods used to eliminate or reduce the transmission of infectious organisms is called _____.

    a. transmission control   **c.** organism control

    b. infection reduction   **d.** infection control   ____

72. Different bacteria move in different ways, and self-movement is known as _____.

    a. migration   **c.** evolution

    b. motility   **d.** locomotion   ____

73. _____ is an abnormal condition of all or part of the body, or its systems or organs, which makes the body incapable of carrying on normal function.

    a. An allergy   **c.** A disease

    b. An infection   **d.** A contamination   ____

74. Within the field of cosmetology, the ability to produce an effect is known as _____.

    a. effectiveness   **c.** productivity

    b. efficacy   **d.** strength   ____

75. Add _____ when diluting to prevent foaming, which can result in an incorrect mixing ratio.

    a. disinfectant to water

    b. tongs to water

    c. water to disinfectant

    d. draining basket to disinfectant   ____

CHAPTER 6 GENERAL ANATOMY & PHYSIOLOGY

1. The basic units of all living things, from bacteria to plants to animals, including human beings, are _____.
   a. organs
   b. cells
   c. muscles
   d. nerves
   ____

2. The dense, active protoplasm found in the center of the cell is the _____.
   a. cytoplasm
   b. cell membrane
   c. nucleus
   d. chromatid
   ____

3. Mitosis is the usual process of cell reproduction of human tissues that occurs when the cell divides into two identical cells called _____.
   a. mother cells
   b. daughter cells
   c. father cells
   d. son cells
   ____

4. The _____ is the watery fluid that surrounds the nucleus of the cell and is needed for growth, reproduction, and self-repair.
   a. cystine
   b. neuron
   c. cytoplasm
   d. mandible
   ____

5. The study of the functions and activities performed by the body's structures is called _____.
   a. physiology
   b. biology
   c. anatomy
   d. physiography
   ____

6. Structures composed of specialized tissues designed to perform specific functions in plants and animals are known as _____.
   a. tissues
   b. nerves
   c. membranes
   d. organs
   ____

7. Which type of tissue contracts and moves various parts of the body?
   a. Nerve tissue
   b. Muscle tissue
   c. Connective tissue
   d. Epithelial tissue
   ____

8. Which type of tissue lines the heart, digestive and respiratory organs, and the glands?
   - **a.** Nerve tissue
   - **b.** Muscle tissue
   - **c.** Connective tissue
   - **d.** Epithelial tissue ____

9. The connection between two or more bones of the skeleton is called a _____.
   - **a.** ligament
   - **b.** joint
   - **c.** tendon
   - **d.** muscle ____

10. The _____ is the larger of the two bones that form the leg below the knee.
    - **a.** patella
    - **b.** fibula
    - **c.** tibia
    - **d.** femur ____

11. The oval, bony case that protects the brain is the _____.
    - **a.** cranium
    - **b.** facial skeleton
    - **c.** hyoid bone
    - **d.** skull ____

12. The maxillae are the bones of the _____.
    - **a.** lower jaw
    - **b.** upper jaw
    - **c.** upper arm
    - **d.** forearm ____

13. The two bones that form the sides and top of the cranium are the _____.
    - **a.** parietal bones
    - **b.** occipital bones
    - **c.** lacrimal bones
    - **d.** zygomatic bones ____

14. The inner and larger bone in the forearm that is attached to the wrist and located on the side of the little finger is the _____.
    - **a.** carpus
    - **b.** ulna
    - **c.** metacarpus
    - **d.** radius ____

15. The foot is made up of _____ bones.
    - **a.** 6
    - **b.** 11
    - **c.** 18
    - **d.** 26 ____

16. What is the U-shaped bone at the base of the tongue that supports the tongue and its muscles?
    - **a.** Hyoid bone
    - **b.** Masseter
    - **c.** Thorax
    - **d.** Cervical vertebrae ____

17. The part of the muscle that does not move and is attached closest to the skeleton is the _____.
   a. belly   **c.** origin
   b. insertion   **d.** tendon   ____

18. The broad muscle that covers the top of the skull and consists of the occipitalis and frontalis is the

_____.
   a. epicranial aponeurosis
   b. epicranius
   c. sternocleidomastoideus
   d. temporalis   ____

19. The _____ are the muscles that straighten the wrist, hand, and fingers to form a straight line.
   a. extensors   **c.** supinators
   b. pronators   **d.** flexors   ____

20. The muscles that draw a body part, such as a finger, arm, or toe, inward toward the median axis of the body or of an extremity are the _____.
   a. flexors   **c.** extensors
   b. abductors   **d.** adductors   ____

21. The system of nerves that carries impulses, or messages, to and from the central nervous system is called the

_____.
   a. involuntary nervous system
   b. voluntary nervous system
   c. autonomic nerve system
   d. peripheral nervous system   ____

22. Sensory nerve endings called _____ are located close to the surface of the skin.
   a. reactors   **c.** capillaries
   b. receptors   **d.** aural neurons   ____

23. The largest artery in the human body is the _____.
   a. jugular   **c.** aorta
   b. ventricle   **d.** carotid   ____

24. The main blood supply of the arms and hands are the

_____.
   a. facial and superficial arteries
   b. ulnar and radial arteries
   c. radial and posterior arteries
   d. ulnar and external jugular arteries   ____

25. The popliteal artery supplies blood to the foot and divides into two separate arteries known as the _____.
   a. anterior tibial and posterior tibial arteries
   b. anterior tibial and dorsalis pedis arteries
   c. internal and external jugular arteries
   d. supraorbital and infraorbital arteries ____

26. The _____ muscle is the primary nasal muscle of concern to cosmetologists.
   a. buccinator   **c.** risorius
   b. procerus   **d.** triangularis ____

27. The muscle that raises the angle of the mouth and draws it inward is the _____ muscle.
   a. depressor labii inferioris
   b. orbicularis oris
   c. levator anguli oris
   d. levator labii superioris ____

28. The _____ cranial nerve is the chief motor nerve of the face.
   a. fourth   **c.** sixth
   b. fifth   **d.** seventh ____

29. The muscle that covers the back of the neck and the upper and middle region of the back is the _____.
   a. trapezius   **c.** serratus anterior
   b. pectoralis major   **d.** latissimus dorsi ____

30. The median nerve is a sensory-motor nerve that, with its branches, supplies the _____.
   a. fingers and toes   **c.** arm and hand
   b. hand and wrist   **d.** arm and wrist ____

31. The deep peroneal nerve extends down the _____, behind the muscles.
   a. front of the arm   **c.** back of the leg
   b. front of the leg   **d.** back of the arm ____

32. The simplest form of nervous activity that includes a sensory and motor nerve is called a _____.
   a. spasm   **c.** reflex
   b. twitch   **d.** contraction ____

33. Deoxygenated blood flows from the heart to the lungs for oxygenation and waste removal and then returns that blood to the _____ so oxygen-rich blood can be delivered to the body.
    a. left atrium
    c. left ventricle
    b. right atrium
    d. right ventricle ____

34. Which nerve affects the muscles of the mouth?
    a. Temporal
    c. Mandibular
    b. Auricular
    d. Buccal ____

35. Blood _____ the body's temperature.
    a. has no effect upon
    b. helps to equalize
    c. is the only factor affecting
    d. is only capable of raising ____

36. The _____ supplies blood to the muscles of the eye.
    a. inferior labial artery
    c. infraorbital artery
    b. infraorbital nerve
    d. intratrochlear nerve ____

37. The technical term for the facial artery is the _____ artery.
    a. internal maxillary
    c. submental
    b. external maxillary
    d. inferior labial ____

38. The endocrine glands, also known as _____ glands, release hormonal secretions directly into the bloodstream.
    a. ductless
    c. duct
    b. secretory
    d. oil ____

39. Which gland affects almost every physiologic process of the body?
    a. Exocrine
    c. Endocrine
    b. Adrenal
    d. Pituitary ____

40. The _____ nerve supplies impulses to the skin of the forehead, upper eyelids, and interior portion of the scalp, orbit, eyeball, and nasal passage.
    a. mandibular
    c. ophthalmic
    b. maxillary
    d. temporal ____

41. The heart is the organ that keeps the _____ moving within the circulatory system.
    a. lymph   **c.** water
    b. blood   **d.** spinal fluid   ____

42. The complex system that serves as a protective covering and helps regulate the body's temperature is the _____ system.
    a. integumentary   **c.** circulatory
    b. skeletal   **d.** muscular   ____

43. The gastrointestinal system consists of the _____, stomach, intestines, salivary and gastric glands, and other organs.
    a. kidneys   **c.** appendix
    b. liver   **d.** mouth   ____

44. The _____ system distributes blood throughout the body.
    a. integumentary   **c.** respiratory
    b. circulatory   **d.** lymphatic   ____

45. The _____ system is responsible for breaking down foods into nutrients and wastes.
    a. lymphatic   **c.** integumentary
    b. endocrine   **d.** digestive   ____

46. The _____ system is the body system consisting of a group of specialized glands that affect the growth, development, sexual functions, and health of the entire body.
    a. endocrine   **c.** digestive
    b. excretory   **d.** reproductive   ____

47. The _____ system protects the body from disease by developing immunities and destroying disease-causing microorganisms.
    a. skeletal   **c.** endocrine
    b. respiratory   **d.** lymphatic   ____

48. The _____ system covers, shapes, and holds the skeletal system in place.
    a. lymphatic   **c.** nervous
    b. muscular   **d.** integumentary   ____

49. The _____ system controls and coordinates all other systems of the body and makes them work harmoniously and efficiently.
- **a.** lymphatic
- **b.** endocrine
- **c.** integumentary
- **d.** nervous

____

50. The _____ system performs the function of producing offspring and passing on the genetic code from one generation to another.
- **a.** reproductive
- **b.** genetic
- **c.** hereditary
- **d.** familial

____

51. The _____ system makes blood and oxygen available to body structures through breathing and eliminating carbon dioxide.
- **a.** nervous
- **b.** reproductive
- **c.** respiratory
- **d.** endocrine

____

52. The _____ system forms the physical foundation of the body.
- **a.** skeletal
- **b.** muscular
- **c.** nervous
- **d.** reproductive

____

53. The study of the human body structures that can be seen with the naked eye and how the body parts are organized is _____.
- **a.** physiology
- **b.** histology
- **c.** mycology
- **d.** anatomy

____

54. Neurology is the scientific study of the structure, function, and pathology of the _____.
- **a.** muscular system
- **b.** integumentary system
- **c.** skeletal system
- **d.** nervous system

____

55. Lymph nodes filter the _____ vessels, which helps fight infection.
- **a.** platelet
- **b.** lymphatic
- **c.** blood
- **d.** plasma

____

CHAPTER 7 SKIN STRUCTURE, GROWTH, & NUTRITION

1. A physician who specializes in diseases and disorders of the skin, hair, and nails is _____.
   a. a histologist
   b. a dermatologist
   c. an esthetician
   d. a pediatrician _____

2. Healthy skin has _____ texture and is smooth.
   a. a fine-grained
   b. a dry
   c. a rough
   d. an inflexible _____

3. Appendages of the skin include hair, nails, and sudoriferous and _____ glands.
   a. sebaceous
   b. endocrine
   c. adrenal
   d. exocrine _____

4. Which of the following correctly identifies the layers of skin and fat from the outermost layer to the innermost layer?
   a. Dermis, subcutaneous, epidermis
   b. Epidermis, subcutaneous, dermis
   c. Dermis, epidermis, subcutaneous
   d. Epidermis, dermis, subcutaneous _____

5. As cells die they are pushed to the surface to replace dead cells that are shed from the _____.
   a. stratum corneum
   b. stratum lucidum
   c. stratum germinativum
   d. stratum granulosum _____

6. The layer directly beneath the epidermis is the _____.
   a. reticular layer
   b. stratum spinosum
   c. papillary layer
   d. subcutaneous tissue _____

7. Which type of tissue gives smoothness and contour to the body, contains fats for use as energy, and also acts as a protective cushion for the skin?
   a. Subcutaneous tissue
   b. Cardiac tissue
   c. Muscle tissue
   d. Nerve tissue _____

8. Which nerve fibers are distributed to the arrector pili muscles attached to the hair follicles?
   a. Impulse nerve fibers
   b. Sensory nerve fibers
   c. Secretory nerve fibers
   d. Motor nerve fibers _____

9. Nerves that regulate the excretion of perspiration from the sudoriferous glands and control the flow of sebum to the surface of the skin are _____.
   a. motor nerve fibers
   b. sensory nerve fibers
   c. secretory nerve fibers
   d. impulse nerve fibers ____

10. _____ fibers react to heat, cold, touch, pressure, and pain.
   a. Motor nerve
   b. Sensory nerve
   c. Secretory nerve
   d. Complex nerve ____

11. The amount and type of pigment produced in an individual is determined by his or her _____.
   a. genes
   b. gender
   c. sun exposure
   d. age ____

12. Skin gets its strength, form, and flexibility from _____.
   a. collagen and keratin
   b. sebum and melanin
   c. keratin and elastin
   d. collagen and elastin ____

13. The sudoriferous glands excrete perspiration, detoxify the body, and _____.
   a. preserve the softness of the hair
   b. lubricate the skin
   c. produce collagen
   d. regulate body temperature ____

14. To keep your body healthy, you must be sure that what you eat helps to _____.
   a. prevent hydration
   b. cause fatigue
   c. delay the rate of aging
   d. regulate the overall function of your cells ____

15. Which vitamin aids in and accelerates the skin's healing processes and is vitally important in fighting the aging process?
   a. Vitamin A
   b. Vitamin C
   c. Vitamin D
   d. Vitamin E ____

16. The epidermis is the _____ layer of the skin.
   a. healthiest
   b. thickest
   c. thinnest
   d. most important ____

17. The scalp has larger and deeper _____ than the skin on the rest of the body.
    a. melanocytes
    b. Propionibacterium acnes
    c. sensory nerve fibers
    d. hair follicles ____

18. During excretion, perspiration from the _____ glands is excreted through the skin.
    a. sudoriferous
    b. sebaceous
    c. reticular
    d. papillary ____

19. One of the best ways to follow a healthy diet is to read _____.
    a. magazine articles
    b. food labels
    c. diet books
    d. legal guidelines ____

20. Emotional stress and hormone imbalances can increase the flow of _____.
    a. sebum
    b. spinal fluid
    c. lymph
    d. pus ____

21. The nutrient needed for energy to run every function within the body is _____.
    a. vitamins
    b. proteins
    c. carbohydrates
    d. fats ____

22. The USDA recommends that people eat _____.
    a. zero salt and zero sugar
    b. large amounts of salt and sugar
    c. moderate amounts of salt and sugar
    d. moderate amounts of salt and no sugar ____

23. Vitamins are considered _____.
    a. nutritional requirements
    b. nutritional supplements
    c. cosmetic ingredients
    d. prescription medications ____

24. Water makes up _____ percent of the body's weight and is necessary for virtually every function of the cells and body.
    a. 10–20
    b. 20–30
    c. 30–50
    d. 50–70 ____

25. Lack of water is the principal cause of _____.
    a. daytime fatigue
    b. daytime hunger
    c. daytime mood swings
    d. daytime memory loss ____

26. Small, cone-shaped elevations at the base of the hair follicles are _____.
   a. melanocytes
   b. papules
   c. dermal papillae
   d. secretory coils
   ____

27. The layer of the epidermis where the process of skin cell shedding begins is the _____.
   a. stratum corneum
   b. stratum lucidum
   c. stratum germinativum
   d. stratum spinosum
   ____

28. The coiled base of the sudoriferous gland is known as the _____.
   a. secretory coil
   b. sweat duct
   c. sebaceous gland
   d. elastin coil
   ____

29. A small elevation on the skin that contains no fluid but may develop pus is a _____.
   a. comedo
   b. papule
   c. callus
   d. pustule
   ____

30. Fatty tissue found below the dermis is _____ tissue.
   a. secretory
   b. sudoriferous
   c. subcutaneous
   d. sensory
   ____

31. A raised, inflamed papule with a white or yellow center containing pus in the top of the lesion is a _____.
   a. papillary
   b. pustule
   c. callus
   d. comedo
   ____

32. The outer layer of the epidermis is the _____ layer.
   a. stratum corneum
   b. stratum granulosum
   c. stratum lucidum
   d. stratum germinativum
   ____

33. The clear, transparent layer of the epidermis under the stratum corneum is the _____.
   a. stratum spinosum
   b. stratum granulosum
   c. stratum germinativum
   d. stratum lucidum
   ____

34. A fatty or oily secretion that lubricates the skin and preserves the softness of the hair is _____.
   a. sebum
   b. lymph
   c. pus
   d. melanin
   ____

35. The layer of the epidermis also known as the basal cell layer is the _____.
   a. stratum lucidum
   b. stratum spinosum
   c. stratum corneum
   d. stratum germinativum
   ____

8 SKIN DISORDERS & DISEASES

1. Many scientists and dermatologists believe that extrinsic factors such as exposure to the sun or smoking are responsible for up to _____ percent of skin aging.
   - **a.** 50
   - **b.** 60
   - **c.** 75
   - **d.** 85 _____

2. It is recommended that you wear a broad-spectrum sunscreen with an SPF of at least _____ on a daily basis.
   - **a.** 5
   - **b.** 8
   - **c.** 15
   - **d.** 30 _____

3. A _____ is an abnormal, rounded, solid lump above, within, or under the skin that is larger than a papule.
   - **a.** tubercle
   - **b.** mole
   - **c.** macula
   - **d.** bulla _____

4. Which of these terms refers to thin, dry, or oily plates of epidermal flakes?
   - **a.** Fissures
   - **b.** Keloids
   - **c.** Pustules
   - **d.** Scales _____

5. Benign, keratin-filled cysts that appear just under the epidermis and have no visible openings are _____.
   - **a.** milia
   - **b.** ulcers
   - **c.** crust
   - **d.** pustules _____

6. An open comedo is also known as a _____.
   - **a.** mole
   - **b.** birthmark
   - **c.** blackhead
   - **d.** whitehead _____

7. Which of these is an inflammatory, uncomfortable, and often chronic disease of the skin, characterized by moderate to severe inflammation, scaling, and sometimes severe itching?
   - **a.** Eczema
   - **b.** Acne
   - **c.** Psoriasis
   - **d.** Herpes simplex _____

8. A _____ is an abnormal brown- or wine-colored skin discoloration with a circular or irregular shape.
   a. mole
   c. chloasma
   b. stain
   d. lentigo _____

9. The absence of melanin pigment in the body and skin sensitivity to light are signs of _____.
   a. nevus
   c. asteatosis
   b. lentignes
   d. albinism _____

10. What is the most dangerous form of skin cancer, often characterized by black or dark brown patches on the skin that may appear uneven in texture, jagged, or raised?
    a. Basal cell carcinoma
    b. Malignant melanoma
    c. Squamous cell carcinoma
    d. Verruca cell _____

11. A cosmetologist must not serve a client who is suffering from an inflamed skin disorder, regardless of whether it is infectious, unless the client _____.
    a. needs a facial quickly for an important event such as a wedding
    b. declares that he or she is practicing doctor-prescribed home care
    c. has a physician's note permitting the client to receive services
    d. signs a waiver clearing the cosmetologist and the salon of liability _____

12. A skin condition caused by an inflammation of the sebaceous glands that is often characterized by redness, dry or oily scaling, crusting, and/or itchiness is _____.
    a. contact dermatitis
    b. irritant contact dermatitis
    c. allergic contact dermatitis
    d. seborrheic dermatitis _____

13. The term _____ refers to abnormal colorations that accompany skin disorders and are symptoms of many systemic disorders.
    a. anhidrosis
    c. dyschromias
    b. bromhidrosis
    d. conjunctivitis _____

14. A(n) _____ is a type of keratoma.
- **a.** callus
- **b.** keloid
- **c.** lesion
- **d.** excoriation

_____

15. Acne is a skin disorder characterized by chronic inflammation of the _____ glands.
- **a.** sudoriferous
- **b.** sebaceous
- **c.** sweat
- **d.** adrenaline

_____

16. A predisposition to acne is based on heredity and _____.
- **a.** diet
- **b.** age
- **c.** use of noncomedogenic makeup
- **d.** hormones

_____

17. Noncomedogenic products are specifically designed and proven not to clog the _____.
- **a.** bullas
- **b.** dyschromias
- **c.** follicles
- **d.** sebaceous glands

_____

18. People have _____ over the intrinsic factors that affect skin aging.
- **a.** no control
- **b.** little control
- **c.** considerable control
- **d.** total control

_____

19. The best defense against pollutants is to _____.
- **a.** wear sunscreen whenever you are outside
- **b.** avoid touching your face with your hands
- **c.** follow a good daily skin care routine
- **d.** wear long-sleeved clothing when you are outdoors

_____

20. Irritant contact dermatitis occurs when irritating substances temporarily damage the _____.
- **a.** dermis
- **b.** epidermis
- **c.** papillary layer
- **d.** hair follicles

_____

21. A pustule is a raised, inflamed papule with a white or yellow center containing _____ in the top of the lesion.
- **a.** water
- **b.** blood
- **c.** lymph
- **d.** pus

_____

22. A _____ is a large, protruding pocket-like lesion filled with sebum.
- **a.** closed comedo
- **b.** sebaceous cyst
- **c.** bulla
- **d.** miliaria rubra

_____

23. A flat spot or discoloration on the skin, also known as a "liver" spot, is a _____.
a. macule   c. milia
b. leukoderma   d. scale   ____

24. Foul-smelling perspiration, usually noticeable in the armpits or on the feet, that is generally caused by bacteria is _____.
a. hyperhidrosis   c. anhidrosis
b. miliaria rubra   d. bromhidrosis   ____

25. A _____ is a slightly raised mark on the skin formed after an injury or lesion of the skin has healed.
a. mole   c. scale
b. scar   d. stain   ____

26. A contagious bacterial skin infection characterized by weeping lesions is _____.
a. impetigo   c. eczema
b. conjunctivitis   d. herpes simplex   ____

27. A _____ is an itchy, swollen lesion that lasts only a few hours.
a. wheal   c. verruca
b. vesicle   d. tubercle   ____

28. A(n) _____ is a crack in the skin that penetrates the dermis.
a. ulcer   c. excoriation
b. fissure   d. crust   ____

29. A small blister or sac containing clear fluid, lying within or just beneath the epidermis is a _____.
a. tubercle   c. vesicle
b. tumor   d. wheal   ____

30. A large blister containing a watery fluid that is similar to a vesicle is _____.
a. a tubercule   c. a cyst
b. a macule   d. a bulla   ____

31. In the ABCDE Cancer Checklist established by the American Cancer Society, what does the C stand for?
a. Crust   c. Caliber
b. Color   d. Circumference   ____

32. When bacteria cannot survive in the presence of oxygen, it is known as _____.
    a. anaerobic
    b. anesthetic
    c. hyperkinetic
    d. aerobic
    ____

33. UVA rays, also known as _____, are deep-penetrating rays that can even go through a glass window.
    a. enhancing rays
    b. tanning rays
    c. aging rays
    d. burning rays
    ____

34. An allergic reaction created by repeated exposure to a chemical or a substance is known as _____.
    a. contact irritation
    b. sensitization
    c. non-contact irritation
    d. irritant contact dermatitis
    ____

35. An acute inflammatory disorder of the sweat glands, characterized by the eruption of small, red vesicles and accompanied by burning, itching skin is _____
    a. hyperhidrosis
    b. miliaria rubra
    c. anhidrosis
    d. bromhidrosia
    ____

9 NAIL STRUCTURE & GROWTH

1. A normal, healthy nail surface _____.
   a. is completely inflexible   **c.** is shiny and smooth
   b. has a spotted surface   **d.** is white and opaque   ____

2. The portion of the living skin that supports the nail plate as it grows toward the free edge is called the _____.
   a. nail bed   **c.** matrix
   b. cuticle   **d.** ligament   ____

3. The _____ is the whitish, half-moon shape underneath the base of the nail.
   a. sidewall   **c.** root
   b. lunula   **d.** free edge   ____

4. The part of the nail plate that extends over the tip of the finger or toe is the _____.
   a. free edge   **c.** bed epithelium
   b. matrix   **d.** sidewall   ____

5. A _____ is a tough band of fibrous tissue that connects bones or holds an organ in place.
   a. muscle   **c.** tendon
   b. ligament   **d.** nerve   ____

6. The _____ is the fold of skin overlapping the side of the nail.
   a. eponychium   **c.** nail groove
   b. hyponychium   **d.** sidewall   ____

7. As long as the _____ is nourished and healthy, new nail plate cells will be created.
   a. lateral nail fold   **c.** matrix
   b. lunula   **d.** nail plate   ____

8. Ordinarily, replacement of a natural fingernail takes about _____.
   a. six to twelve months   **c.** six to eight months
   b. four to six months   **d.** two to eight months   ____

9. The nail growth rate on the _____ is typically the slowest.
   a. thumb
   b. middle finger
   c. pinkie finger
   d. index finger
   ____

10. The nail has a water content between _____.
   a. 10 and 15 percent
   b. 1 and 5 percent
   c. 20 and 45 percent
   d. 15 and 25 percent
   ____

11. The natural nail is an appendage of the _____.
   a. dermis
   b. epidermis
   c. skin
   d. skeletal system
   ____

12. The appearance of the nails can reflect the general health of the _____.
   a. body
   b. skin
   c. muscular system
   d. skeletal system
   ____

13. The _____ is relatively porous and will allow water to pass through it.
   a. nail bed
   b. matrix
   c. nail plate
   d. eponychium
   ____

14. The matrix contains _____.
   a. muscles and blood vessels
   b. nerves, lymph, and blood vessels
   c. water and muscles
   d. water, ligaments, and blood vessels
   ____

15. Tissue that adheres directly to the natural nail plate but which can be removed with gentle scraping is the _____.
   a. perionychium
   b. hyponychium
   c. eponychium
   d. cuticle
   ____

16. Cosmetologists are allowed to gently _____ the eponychium.
   a. cut
   b. trim
   c. push back
   d. file
   ____

17. Cuticle moisturizers, softeners, and conditioners are actually designed for the eponychium, _____, and hyponychium.
   a. cuticle
   b. nail plate
   c. lateral sidewalls
   d. lunula
   ____

46

18. Toenails are thicker than fingernails because the
_____ of the toenail is longer than that of the
fingernail.

    a. nail bed   **c.** lunula

    b. matrix   **d.** eponychium   ____

19. Unlike healthy hair, healthy nails are not _____
periodically.

    a. cut   **c.** shed

    b. cleaned   **d.** maintained   ____

20. It takes about _____ for toenails to be fully
replaced.

    a. three to six months

    b. six to nine months

    c. nine to twelve months

    d. twelve to fifteen months   ____

21. The living skin at the base of the natural nail plate covering
the matrix area is the _____.

    a. eponychium   **c.** cuticle

    b. hyponychium   **d.** lunula   ____

22. The thin layer of tissue that attaches the nail plate and the
nail bed is the _____.

    a. bed eponychium   **c.** lateral nail fold

    b. bed epithelium   **d.** onyx   ____

23. The slightly thickened layer of skin under the nail that lies
between the fingertip and the free edge of the nail plate is
the _____.

    a. epithelium   **c.** sidewall

    b. eponychium   **d.** hyponychium   ____

24. The dead, colorless tissue attached to the natural nail plate
is known as the nail _____.

    a. bed   **c.** groove

    b. fold   **d.** cuticle   ____

25. The _____ is the area where the nail plate cells are
formed.

    a. cuticle   **c.** matrix

    b. lunula   **d.** free edge   ____

CHAPTER 10 NAIL DISORDERS & DISEASES

1. A normal, healthy nail is firm but flexible and should be
   _____.
   a. smooth and unspotted
   b. uneven with few ridges
   c. long with a satin finish
   d. short and opaque   ____

2. If a client has ridges running vertically down the length
   of the natural nail plate, it is recommended that you
   _____.
   a. aggressively file the nail plate   c. thin the nail plate
   b. carefully buff the nail plate   d. remove the free edge   ____

3. The medical term for fungal infections of the feet is
   _____.
   a. tinea pathogenic   c. tinea alopecia
   b. tinea pedis   d. paronychia   ____

4. A typical pseudomonal bacterial infection on the nail plate
   can be identified in the early stages as a _____
   spot that becomes darker in its advanced stages.
   a. orange-red   c. blue-green
   b. white-gray   d. light-green

5. The separation and falling off of a nail plate from the nail
   bed is _____.
   a. onychia   c. onychomadesis
   b. paronychia   d. pyogenic granuloma   ____

6. Onychorrhexis is caused by injury to the matrix, excessive
   use of cuticle removers, harsh cleaning agents, aggressive
   filing techniques, or _____.
   a. illness   c. allergies
   b. heredity   d. improper nutrition   ____

7. Tiny pits or severe roughness on the surface of the nail
   plate are signs of which condition?
   a. Paronychia   c. Nail psoriasis
   b. Onychocryptosis   d. Onychomycosis   ____

8. The term _____ refers to a condition caused by injury, heredity, or previous disease of the nail unit.
   a. nail psoriasis
   c. nail disorder
   b. nail pterygium
   d. nail disease
   ____

9. Splinter hemorrhages are caused by physical trauma or injury to the _____.
   a. nail plate
   c. free edge
   b. nail bed
   d. lunula
   ____

10. Nail fungi are contagious and can be transmitted through _____ instruments.
    a. sterilized
    c. contaminated
    b. disinfected
    d. disposable
    ____

11. Onychomadesis can usually be traced to a localized infection, injuries to the matrix, or _____.
    a. a severe systemic illness
    c. mild allergies
    b. an external medications
    d. a split fingernail
    ____

12. Any deformity or disease of the natural nail is known as _____.
    a. onychauxis
    c. onychia
    b. onychosis
    d. paronychia
    ____

13. Which condition is characterized by nail plates that are noticeably thin, white, and more flexible than normal?
    a. Melanonychia
    c. Agnail
    b. Plicatured nail
    d. Eggshell nails
    ____

14. Which of the following is a common cause of surface stains on nails?
    a. Nail polish remover
    c. Smoking
    b. Allergies
    d. Poor blood circulation
    ____

15. The condition in which a blood clot forms under the nail plate, causing a dark purplish spot, is _____.
    a. discolored nails
    c. blue fingernails
    b. bruised nail beds
    d. plicatured nails
    ____

16. The condition in which the living skin around the nail splits and tears is _____.
    a. a hangnail
    c. melanonychia
    b. Beau's lines
    d. onychophagy
    ____

17. The lifting of the nail plate from the bed without shedding is
_____.
   a. onychosis
   b. onychocryptosis
   c. onycholysis
   d. onychomadesis _____

18. The term _____ refers to darkening of the fingernails or toenails.
   a. melanonychia
   b. nail pterygium
   c. paronychia
   d. splinter hemorrhages _____

19. When increased crosswise curvature throughout the nail plate results in the free edge pinching the sidewalls into a deep curve, it is known as pincer nail or _____.
   a. bruised nail
   b. circular nail
   c. eggshell nail
   d. trumpet nail _____

20. Visible depressions running across the width of the natural nail plate are known as _____.
   a. ridges
   b. splinters
   c. Beau's lines
   d. agnail _____

21. Blue fingernails are usually caused by a lack of _____ in the red blood cells.
   a. leukocytes
   b. circulating oxygen
   c. water
   d. melanin _____

22. Koilonychia are soft spoon nails with a _____ shape.
   a. convex
   b. concave
   c. elongated
   d. curved _____

23. The technical term for white spots, or whitish discolorations of the nails is _____.
   a. leukonychia spots
   b. albinism
   c. melanonychia spots
   d. pigment disorder _____

24. The technical term for bitten nails is _____.
   a. onychorrhexis
   b. plicatured nails
   c. onychophagy
   d. onycholysis _____

25. An abnormal condition that occurs when the skin is stretched by the nail plate is _____.
   a. onychogryposis
   b. claw nails
   c. ram's horn
   d. nail pterygium _____

26. A fungal infection of the natural nail plate is known as
_____.

    a. onychomycosis   **c.** onychogryposis
    b. onychia   **d.** paronychia   ____

27. A severe inflammation of the nail in which a lump of red
tissue grows up from the nail bed to the nail plate is known
as _____.

    a. tinea pedis   **c.** paronychia
    b. pyogenic granuloma   **d.** onychorrhexis   ____

28. The technical term for ingrown nails is _____.

    a. nail psoriasis   **c.** onychocryptosis
    b. onychorrhexis   **d.** onychophagy   ____

29. A proper hand analysis will allow you to identify disease,
disorders, and conditions, including signs of infection,
which may be identified through pain, redness, swelling
throbbing, and _____.

    a. texture   **c.** moisture level
    b. pus   **d.** scar tissue   ____

30. After performing the nail examination, you should identify
any form of onychosis, note the apparent cause, suggest
the proper service or refer the client to a physician, and
_____.

    a. discuss home maintenance and a future service plan
    b. discuss scheduling the next appointment
    c. schedule treatment for onychosis
    d. thank the client for her time   ____

CHAPTER 11 PROPERTIES OF THE HAIR & SCALP

1. The scientific study of hair, its diseases, and care is called
   _____.
   - **a.** dermatology
   - **b.** trichology
   - **c.** biology
   - **d.** cosmetology   ____

2. The two parts of a mature strand of human hair are the
   _____.
   - **a.** dermis and epidermis
   - **b.** hair shaft and hair follicle
   - **c.** hair root and hair shaft
   - **d.** hair root and hair follicle ____

3. The tube-like depression or pocket in the skin or scalp that contains the hair root is the _____.
   - **a.** hair follicle
   - **b.** hair shaft
   - **c.** hair bulb
   - **d.** scalp   ____

4. Hair follicles are *not* found on the _____.
   - **a.** forehead area
   - **b.** backs of the hands
   - **c.** soles of the feet
   - **d.** back of the neck   ____

5. The _____ is the small, involuntary muscle in the base of the hair follicle.
   - **a.** medulla
   - **b.** arrector pili muscle
   - **c.** tinea
   - **d.** dermal papilla   ____

6. The fatty or oily substance secreted by the sebaceous glands is _____.
   - **a.** sweat
   - **b.** lymph
   - **c.** catagen
   - **d.** sebum   ____

7. For chemicals to penetrate a healthy cuticle hair layer, they must have _____.
   - **a.** no pH
   - **b.** a neutral pH
   - **c.** an alkaline pH
   - **d.** an acidic pH   ____

8. The medulla is composed of _____ cells.
   - **a.** rod-shaped
   - **b.** round
   - **c.** spiral-shaped
   - **d.** rectangular   ____

9. During the _____ phase, new hair is produced because new cells are actively manufactured in the hair follicle.
   a. anagen
   b. catagen
   c. resting
   d. telogen

   ___

10. The major elements that make up human hair are carbon, oxygen, hydrogen, _____.
    a. lead, and zinc
    b. keratin, and selenium
    c. boron, and calcium
    d. nitrogen, and sulfur

    ___

11. The strong, chemical bonds that join amino acids are called _____.
    a. convex bonds
    b. peptide bonds
    c. hydrogen bonds
    d. side bonds

    ___

12. Which type of melanin provides natural colors ranging from red and ginger to yellow and blond tones?
    a. Pheomelanin
    b. Eumelanin
    c. Polymelanin
    d. Biomelanin

    ___

13. Asians tend to have _____ hair.
    a. extremely straight
    b. extremely curly
    c. straight to wavy
    d. wavy to curly

    ___

14. To help minimize tangles in extremely curly hair when shampooing, you should use _____.
    a. a drying shampoo
    b. strong scalp manipulations
    c. a detangling rinse
    d. antibacterial shampoo

    ___

15. Hair texture is classified as _____.
    a. wavy, straight, or curly
    b. coarse, medium, or fine
    c. light, medium, or dark
    d. long, medium, or short

    ___

16. The measurement of the number of individual hair strands on one square inch (2.5 square centimeters) of the scalp is _____.
    a. hair density
    b. hair elasticity
    c. hair texture
    d. hair porosity

    ___

17. Compared to hair with high porosity, chemical services performed on hair with low porosity require _____.
    a. neutral solutions
    b. more acidic solutions
    c. solutions of the same pH
    d. more alkaline solutions

    ___

18. Wet hair with normal elasticity will stretch up to
    _____ of its original length and return to that length
    without breaking.
    a. 25 percent   c. 50 percent
    b. 40 percent   d. 70 percent   _____

19. Oily hair and scalp can be treated by properly washing with
    a _____.
    a. vinegar solution   c. conditioning shampoo
    b. normalizing shampoo d. dry shampoo   _____

20. Which type of hair almost never has a medulla?
    a. Oily   c. Terminal
    b. Pigmented   d. Vellus   _____

21. During which phase does the follicle canal shrink and
    detach from the dermal papilla?
    a. Patagen   c. Anagen
    b. Telogen   d. Catagen   _____

22. The average growth of healthy scalp hair is _____.
    a. ½ inch (1.25 centimeters) per week
    b. 1 inch (2.5 centimeters) per week
    c. ½ inch (1.25 centimeters) per month
    d. 1 inch (2.5 centimeters) per month   _____

23. The technical term used to describe gray hair is
    _____.
    a. canities   c. alopecia
    b. tinea   d. albino   _____

24. A condition of abnormal growth of terminal hair in
    areas of the body that normally grow only vellus hair is
    _____.
    a. trichorrhexis   c. hypertrichosis
    b. ringed hair   d. canities   _____

25. The technical term for dandruff is _____.
    a. canities   c. alopecia
    b. pityriasis   d. simplex   _____

26. Which of the five main structures of the hair root contain the
    blood and nerve supply that provides the nutrients needed
    for hair growth?
    a. Dermal papilla   c. Hair follicle
    b. Hair bulb   d. Sebaceous glands   _____

27. Because there are so many of them, salt bonds account for about _____ of the hair's overall strength.
    a. one quarter
    b. one half
    c. one third
    d. two thirds
    ____

28. The anagen phase generally lasts from three to five

    _____.
    a. days
    b. weeks
    c. months
    d. years
    ____

29. Scalp hair grows _____ on women than on men.
    a. slower
    b. faster
    c. thinner
    d. thicker
    ____

30. The _____ phase signals the end of the growth phase.
    a. telogen
    b. resting
    c. anagen
    d. catagen
    ____

31. Scalp massage _____ hair growth.
    a. increases
    b. decreases
    c. does not increase
    d. is necessary for
    ____

32. Compared to pigmented hair, gray hair is _____.
    a. exactly the same
    b. softer
    c. more resistant
    d. less resistant
    ____

33. Cross-sections of hair _____.
    a. are always round
    b. are always oval
    c. are always flattened oval
    d. can be almost any shape
    ____

34. Bald men are commonly perceived as _____.
    a. more assertive
    b. younger
    c. more physically attractive
    d. less successful
    ____

35. By age 35, almost _____ percent of both men and women show some degree of hair loss.
    a. 20
    b. 30
    c. 40
    d. 50
    ____

36. Finasteride is an oral prescription medication for hair loss that is meant for _____.
   a. men only   c. men and women
   b. women only   d. animals   ____

37. Congenital canities exists _____.
   a. at or before birth   c. during middle age
   b. during adolescence   d. in the later years of life   ____

38. Dandruff can easily be mistaken for _____.
   a. tinea   c. pediculosis capitis
   b. dry scalp   d. trichoptilosis   ____

39. Current research confirms that dandruff is the result of a _____.
   a. bacterium   c. parasite
   b. virus   d. fungus   ____

40. When the living cells of hair form and begin their journey upward through the hair follicle, they mature in a process called _____.
   a. neutralization   c. keratinization
   b. transition   d. maturation   ____

41. Tinea is characterized by _____, scales, and sometimes, painful circular lesions.
   a. numbness   c. sudden hair loss
   b. blisters   d. itching   ____

42. The infestation of the hair and scalp with head lice is called _____.
   a. hypertrichosis   c. pediculosis capitis
   b. trichoptilosis   d. fragilitas crinium   ____

43. A carbuncle is similar to a furuncle but is _____.
   a. smaller   c. harder
   b. larger   d. softer   ____

44. Fine hair is _____ than coarse or medium hair.
   a. thicker
   b. harder to process
   c. more difficult to damage
   d. more fragile   ____

45. Coarse hair _____.
   a. has the smallest diameter
   b. is the most common hair texture
   c. is not resistant to chemical services
   d. is stronger than fine hair
   ____

46. The _____ is the outermost layer of the hair.
   a. hair cuticle   **c.** hair follicle
   b. hair bulb   **d.** hair root
   ____

47. The oil glands in the skin that are connected to the hair follicles are the _____ glands.
   a. systine   **c.** sebaceous
   b. simplex   **d.** scutula
   ____

48. A _____ bond is a weak, physical, cross-link side bond easily broken by water or heat.
   a. hydrogen   **c.** hydrophobic
   b. hydrophillic   **d.** helix
   ____

49. Hair is approximately _____ percent protein.
   a. 60   **c.** 80
   b. 70   **d.** 90
   ____

50. Total scalp hair loss is known as _____.
   a. alopecia areata   **c.** alopecia totalis
   b. androgenetic alopecia **d.** alopecia universalis
   ____

51. Hypertrichosis is also known as _____.
   a. ringed hair   **c.** canities
   b. hirsuties   **d.** split ends
   ____

52. The naturally occurring fungus that causes the symptoms of dandruff when it grows out of control is _____.
   a. medulla   **c.** malassezia
   b. monilethrix   **d.** hypertrichosis
   ____

53. The _____ is the lowest part of a hair strand.
   a. hair root   **c.** hair cuticle
   b. hair bulb   **d.** hair follicle
   ____

54. The technical term for beaded hair is _____.
   a. monilethrix   **c.** trichorrhexis nodosa
   b. fragilitas crinium   **d.** hypertrichosis
   ____

55. A highly contagious skin disease caused by a parasite called a mite that burrows under the skin is _____.
   a. capitis
   b. scabies
   c. furuncle
   d. carbuncle

   ____

56. The term for the spiral shape of a coiled protein is _____.
   a. matrix
   b. cystine
   c. helix
   d. cysteine

   ____

57. Shaving, clipping, and cutting the hair on the head _____.
   a. makes it grow back faster
   b. makes it grow back darker
   c. makes it grow back coarser
   d. has no effect on hair growth

   ____

58. Dry, sulfur-yellow, cuplike crusts on the scalp are called _____.
   a. tinea barbae
   b. scabies
   c. scutula
   d. wheals

   ____

59. The _____ are part of the integumentary system.
   a. hair, skin, and bones
   b. hair, skin, nails, and glands
   c. hair, glands, and bones
   d. nails, skin, and muscles

   ____

60. The long, coarse, pigmented hair found on the scalp, legs, arms, and bodies of males and females is called _____.
   a. vellus hair
   b. lanugo hair
   c. extra hair
   d. terminal hair

   ____

61. The technical term for knotted hair is _____.
   a. trichorrhexis nodosa
   b. monilethrix
   c. trichoptilosis
   d. hypertrichosis

   ____

62. The _____ is the innermost layer of the hair and is composed of round cells.
   a. tinea
   b. monilethrix
   c. medulla
   d. scutula

   ____

63. When hair leaves the follicles at an angle and forms patterns or streams on the head, it is called _____.
    - **a.** crown hair
    - **b.** a cowlick
    - **c.** ringed hair
    - **d.** a whorl

    ____

64. The part of the hair located below the surface of the epidermis is the _____.
    - **a.** hair root
    - **b.** hair shaft
    - **c.** hair stream
    - **d.** hair bulb

    ____

65. A particular pattern of hair stream that is usually more noticeable on the front hairline in people with short, thick hair is a _____.
    - **a.** cystine
    - **b.** cysteine
    - **c.** cortex
    - **d.** cowlick

    ____

66. The ability of the hair to absorb moisture is called _____.
    - **a.** hair absorbency
    - **b.** hair porosity
    - **c.** hair saturation
    - **d.** hair stream

    ____

67. The middle layer of the hair is the _____.
    - **a.** cortex
    - **b.** carbuncle
    - **c.** canity
    - **d.** catagen

    ____

68. An autoimmune disorder that causes the affected hair follicles to be mistakenly attacked by a person's own immune system is _____.
    - **a.** androgenic alopecia
    - **b.** alopecia areata
    - **c.** alopecia totalis
    - **d.** alopecia universalis

    ____

69. Vellus hair is also known as _____.
    - **a.** lanugo hair
    - **b.** lanthionine hair
    - **c.** malassezia hair
    - **d.** monilethrix hair

    ____

70. The technical term for ringworm is _____.
    - **a.** tinea
    - **b.** tinea barbae
    - **c.** tinea favosa
    - **d.** tinea capitis

    ____

12 BASICS OF CHEMISTRY

1. Inorganic chemistry is the study of substances that do not contain the element carbon, but may contain which element?
   a. Silicon
   b. Oxygen
   c. Hydrogen
   d. Nitrogen   ____

2. A substance that cannot be broken down into simpler substances without a loss of identity is _____.
   a. a compound
   b. an ion
   c. a molecule
   d. an element   ____

3. Chemically combining two or more atoms in definite proportion forms _____.
   a. an acid
   b. a molecule
   c. a mixture
   d. a solvent   ____

4. A(n) _____ is a stable physical mixture of two or more substances in a solvent.
   a. solution
   b. emulsion
   c. compound
   d. element   ____

5. A(n) _____ is a substance dissolved into a solution.
   a. solvent
   b. alkali
   c. solute
   d. acid   ____

6. Liquids that are not capable of being mixed together to form stable solutions are considered _____.
   a. emulsions
   b. suspensions
   c. miscible
   d. immiscible   ____

7. Unstable physical mixtures of undissolved particles in a liquid are _____.
   a. suspensions
   b. mixtures
   c. solutes
   d. emulsions   ____

8. An unstable physical mixture of two or more immiscible substances plus a special ingredient is _____.
- **a.** a suspension
- **b.** an emulsion
- **c.** a mixture
- **d.** a solution ____

9. A substance that allows oil and water to mix or emulsify is _____.
- **a.** a reducing agent
- **b.** a surfactant
- **c.** an anion
- **d.** a cation ____

10. The tail of a surfactant molecule is oil-loving or _____.
- **a.** miscible
- **b.** immiscible
- **c.** lipophilic
- **d.** hydrophilic ____

11. An atom or molecule that carries an electrical charge is called an _____.
- **a.** alkaline
- **b.** acid
- **c.** atom
- **d.** ion ____

12. Alpha hydroxy acids (AHAs) are derived from _____ and used in the salon to exfoliate the skin and to help adjust the pH of certain products.
- **a.** plants
- **b.** chemicals
- **c.** minerals
- **d.** food sources ____

13. Chemical reactions that release a significant amount of heat under certain circumstances are _____.
- **a.** endothermic
- **b.** exothermic
- **c.** negative
- **d.** positive ____

14. A substance that has a pH below 7.0 is considered to be _____.
- **a.** combustible
- **b.** neutral
- **c.** acidic
- **d.** alkaline ____

15. Alkanolamines are often used in place of ammonia because they _____.
- **a.** produce less odor
- **b.** are less expensive
- **c.** have a better texture
- **d.** are more effective ____

16. Which of these is *not* composed of organic chemicals?
- **a.** Pesticides
- **b.** Shampoos
- **c.** Synthetic fabrics
- **d.** Minerals ____

17. Elemental molecules contain two or more _____ of the same element in definite proportions.
   a. atoms
   c. cations
   b. ions
   d. silicones   ____

18. Vapor is _____ that has evaporated into a gas-like state.
   a. an element
   c. a liquid
   b. a solid
   d. a chemical   ____

19. An oxidizing agent is a substance that releases _____.
   a. hydrogen
   c. oxygen
   b. nitrogen
   d. carbon   ____

20. A pure substance is a chemical combination of matter in _____ proportions.
   a. unequal
   c. liquid
   b. fixed
   d. vaporized   ____

21. The glitter in nail polish that can separate from the polish is an example of _____.
   a. an emulsion
   c. a solution
   b. a mixture
   d. a suspension   ____

22. Water-in-oil emulsions feel _____ than oil-in-water emulsions.
   a. greasier
   c. wetter
   b. hotter
   d. colder   ____

23. The ingredient used to raise the pH in hair products to allow the solution to penetrate the hair shaft is _____.
   a. an amino acid
   c. an alkaline solution
   b. ammonia
   d. alpha hydroxy acid   ____

24. Volatile organic compounds contain _____ and evaporate very easily.
   a. carbon
   c. oxygen
   b. hydrogen
   d. nitrogen   ____

25. The chemical reaction that combines a substance with oxygen to produce an oxide is _____.
   a. combustion
   c. ionization
   b. oxidation
   d. reduction   ____

26. The term *logarithm* means multiples of _____.
- **a.** 5
- **b.** 10
- **c.** 100
- **d.** 1,000

_____

27. A chemical reaction in which oxidation and reduction take place at the same time is _____.
- **a.** redox
- **b.** oxidization
- **c.** ionization
- **d.** combustion

_____

28. Any substance that occupies space and has mass is _____.
- **a.** an atom
- **b.** an element
- **c.** matter
- **d.** a reaction

_____

29. Characteristics that can only be determined by a chemical reaction and a chemical change in the substance are _____.
- **a.** chemical properties
- **b.** elemental properties
- **c.** molecular properties
- **d.** physical properties

_____

30. A chemical combination of matter in definite proportions is a(n) _____.
- **a.** atomic substance
- **b.** combined substance
- **c.** miscible substance
- **d.** pure substance

_____

31. A physical combination of matter in any proportion is a _____.
- **a.** chemical mixture
- **b.** combined mixture
- **c.** physical mixture
- **d.** pure substance

_____

32. The _____ is the smallest chemical component of an element.
- **a.** anion
- **b.** atom
- **c.** cation
- **d.** molecule

_____

33. Rapid oxidation of a substance accompanied by the production of heat and light is _____.
- **a.** reduction
- **b.** emulsification
- **c.** ionization
- **d.** combustion

_____

34. Characteristics that can be determined without a chemical reaction and that do not involve a chemical change in the substance are _____.
- **a.** chemical properties
- **b.** elemental properties
- **c.** molecular properties
- **d.** physical properties

_____

13 BASICS OF ELECTRICITY

1. The movement of electrons from one atom to another along a conductor is called _____.
   a. an electric charge   **c.** energy flow
   b. electricity   **d.** sparks   ____

2. Electric wires can be covered with a material that does not transmit electricity such as a rubber or plastic coating. This material is known as _____.
   a. an insulator   **c.** a circuit
   b. a conductor   **d.** a fuse   ____

3. An apparatus that changes direct current to alternating current is _____.
   a. a rectifier   **c.** an inverter
   b. a circuit breaker   **d.** a fuse box   ____

4. The term _____ refers to a rapid and interrupted current, flowing first in one direction and then in the opposite direction.
   a. rectifier current   **c.** active current
   b. alternating current   **d.** direct current ____

5. The unit that measures the pressure or force that pushes the electric current forward through a conductor is _____.
   a. an amp   **c.** an ohm
   b. a watt   **d.** a volt   ____

6. Which unit measures the resistance of an electric current?
   a. Ohm   **c.** Amp
   b. Watt   **d.** Volt   ____

7. The device that prevents excessive current from passing through a circuit is called _____.
   a. a fuse   **c.** a kilowatt
   b. a battery   **d.** an ampere   ____

8. A switch that automatically interrupts or shuts off an electric current at the first indication of an overload is _____.

    a. a voltage regulator   **c.** a circuit breaker

    b. an ampere interrupter   **d.** a battery charger   ____

9. The negative electrode of an electrotherapy device is called _____.

    a. an anode   **c.** a carbide

    b. an electron   **d.** a cathode   ____

10. A process that infuses an alkaline product into the tissues from the negative pole toward the positive pole is called _____.

    a. a cataphoresis   **c.** an iontophoresis

    b. an anaphoresis   **d.** a microcurrent   ____

11. Grounding completes _____ and carries the current safely away.

    a. an electric charge   **c.** an electron flow

    b. an electric circuit   **d.** a microcurrent   ____

12. All the electrical appliances you use should _____.

    a. be battery operated

    b. be UL certified

    c. have a two-prong plug

    d. be used near water   ____

13. When using _____, the active electrode is the electrode used on the area to be treated.

    a. alternating current   **c.** electric current

    b. direct current   **d.** galvanic current   ____

14. Microcurrent can be used to _____ and restore elasticity.

    a. decrease metabolism circulation   **c.** reduce lymph

    b. increase muscle tone   **d.** prevent acidic reactions ____

15. Only licensed professionals should use_____.

    a. electric hairdryers equipment   **c.** light therapy

    b. electric steamers   **d.** electric vaporizers   ____

16. A wavelength is the distance between successive peaks of
_____ waves.

   a. electric
   b. electromagnetic

   c. galvanic
   d. infrared   ____

17. Invisible light is the light at either end of the _____
that is invisible to the naked eye.

   a. electromagnetic spectrum
   b. spectrum of radiance

   c. spectrum of radiation
   d. visible spectrum of light   ____

18. Ultraviolet C (UVC) light _____.

   a. is often used in tanning beds
   b. has the longest wavelength
   c. is often called the burning light
   d. is blocked by the ozone layer   ____

19. Catalysts are substances that speed up _____.

   a. chemical reactions
   b. acidic reactions

   c. alkaline reactions
   d. photoxic reactions   ____

20. All lasers work by a process known as selective
_____.

   a. emission
   b. electrolysis

   c. photothermolysis
   d. photosynthesis   ____

21. Constant and direct current, having a positive and negative
pole, which produces chemical changes when it passes
through the tissues and fluids of the body is known as
_____ current.

   a. a galvanic
   b. an alternating

   c. a direct
   d. a conductive   ____

22. An extremely low level of electricity that mirrors the body's
natural electrical impulses is _____.

   a. a minicurrent
   b. a microcurrent

   c. a milliampere
   d. an internal current   ____

23. A medical device that uses multiple colors and wavelengths
of focused light to treat conditions such as excessive hair
and spider veins is _____.

   a. a laser
   b. an infrared light device

   c. an intense pulse light
   d. a light-emitting diode   ____

24. The thermal or heat-producing current with a high rate of oscillation or vibration that is commonly used for scalp and facial treatments is called _____.
    a. a Tesla light-emitting current
    b. an ultraviolet light
    c. an intense pulse light
    d. a Tesla high-frequency current   ____

25. A device that works by releasing light onto the skin to stimulate specific responses at precise depths of the skin tissue is _____.
    a. a laser   c. an intense pulse light
    b. an infrared light device   d. a light-emitting diode   ____

26. For safety, use no more than _____ plug(s) in each outlet.
    a. one   c. three
    b. two   d. four   ____

27. When _____ is heated, it produces positive and negative ions that cancel the electric charges in the hair that cause static electricity.
    a. aluminum   c. tourmaline
    b. stainless steel   d. an insulator   ____

28. The application of UV light must be done with the utmost care in a proper manner by a qualified professional because overexposure can lead to skin _____.
    a. allergies and irritation   c. dryness and scaling
    b. damage and skin cancer   d. excessive sloughing   ____

29. The use of _____ light reduces acne and bacteria on the skin.
    a. green   c. yellow
    b. red   d. blue   ____

30. The unit that measures how much electric energy is being used in one second is _____.
    a. an ohm   c. a watt
    b. a volt   d. an ampere   ____

14 PRINCIPLES OF HAIR DESIGN

MULTIPLE CHOICE

1. Chemically infused services that make changes in the natural texture, curl, or _____ in the hair are considered permanent and will never revert back to the original pattern.
   a. thickness
   b. wave pattern
   c. elasticity
   d. hair color ____

2. For a client with gold skin tones, _____ haircolors are more flattering.
   a. contrasting
   b. toned
   c. warm
   d. cool ____

3. When designing a style for a woman with large hips or broad shoulders, the stylist would normally create a style with _____.
   a. more volume
   b. less volume
   c. more length
   d. darker colors ____

4. Balance is described as establishing equal or appropriate proportions to create _____.
   a. width
   b. symmetry
   c. structure
   d. space ____

5. When the two imaginary halves of a hairstyle have an equal visual weight but are positioned unevenly, the hairstyle is considered to have _____ balance.
   a. horizontal
   b. diagonal
   c. symmetrical
   d. asymmetrical ____

6. A regular pulsation or recurrent pattern of movement in a design is referred to as _____.
   a. rhythm
   b. harmony
   c. focus
   d. balance ____

7. The area in a design where the eye is drawn first before traveling to the rest of the design is called the _____.
   a. balance
   b. axis
   c. emphasis
   d. apex ____

8. To offset or round out the features of a square facial shape, the styling choice is to _____.
   a. create the illusion of width in the forehead
   b. add volume to the sides
   c. make the face seem shorter
   d. create volume between the temples and jaw ____

9. The _____ profile has a receding forehead and chin.
   a. concave   c. straight
   b. circular   d. convex ____

10. The triangular section that begins at the apex, or high point of the head, and ends at the front corners is called the _____.
    a. crown area   c. line area
    b. bang area   d. convex area ____

11. Design texture can be created temporarily with the use of _____.
    a. heat and/or wet styling techniques
    b. cold and/or wet styling techniques
    c. heat and/or dry styling techniques
    d. cold and/or dry styling techniques ____

12. Which of these is not a physical characteristic taken into account when designing an artistic and suitable hairstyle?
    a. Body posture   c. Natural hair color
    b. Facial features   d. Head shape ____

13. Left natural, _____ hair may not support many styling options.
    a. straight, medium   c. straight, fine
    b. straight, coarse   d. wavy, fine ____

14. Which type of hair offers the most versatility in styling?
    a. Wavy, medium hair   c. Wavy, fine hair
    b. Straight, coarse hair   d. Straight, fine hair ____

15. For ease of styling, _____ hair is generally best cut short.
    a. curly, medium
    b. curly, coarse
    c. extremely curly, coarse
    d. very curly, fine ____

16. The _____ profile has a prominent forehead and chin.
    a. concave
    b. convex
    c. straight
    d. wavy   ____

17. For a client with _____, you should direct the hair back and away from the face at the temples.
    a. close-set eyes
    b. a large forehead
    c. a crooked nose
    d. wide-set eyes   ____

18. For a client with a _____, the hair should be directed forward in the chin area.
    a. round jaw
    b. receding chin
    c. small chin
    d. large chin   ____

19. For a client with a _____ nose, bring hair forward at the forehead with softness around the face.
    a. wide, flat
    b. long, narrow
    c. small
    d. prominent   ____

20. If a male client has _____, a fairly close-trimmed beard or even faded beard and mustache would be beneficial to the overall appearance.
    a. dark hair
    b. light hair
    c. a wide face and a large jaw
    d. a wide face and full cheeks ____

21. To create length and height in hair design, use _____ lines.
    a. vertical
    b. horizontal
    c. transitional
    d. single   ____

22. To create width in hair design, use _____ lines.
    a. contrasting
    b. horizontal
    c. diagonal
    d. directional   ____

23. Lines that may move in a clockwise or counter-clockwise direction to create the illusion of movement are _____ lines.
    a. curved
    b. horizontal
    c. single
    d. parallel   ____

24. Repeating lines, known as _____ lines, can be straight or curved.
    a. single
    b. vertical
    c. directional
    d. parallel

    ____

25. Lines with a definite forward or backward movement are _____ lines.
    a. transitional
    b. contrasting
    c. directional
    d. diagonal

    ____

26. The square face shape _____.
    a. is narrow at the temples
    b. has hollow cheeks
    c. is rounded at the jaw
    d. is narrow at the middle third of the face

    ____

27. The face shape featuring a narrow forehead, extreme width through the cheekbones, and a narrow chin is the _____.
    a. inverted-triangle
    b. diamond
    c. heart-shaped
    d. pear-shaped

    ____

28. The _____ face shape features a narrow forehead, wide jaw, and wide chin line.
    a. triangular
    b. oblong
    c. round
    d. square

    ____

29. The face shape featuring a wide forehead and narrow chin line is the _____.
    a. triangular
    b. inverted triangle
    c. oblong
    d. diamond

    ____

30. Which parting is used to create the illusion of width or height in a hairstyle?
    a. Side
    b. Center
    c. Diagonal
    d. Zigzag

    ____

31. The contour and proportions of the _____ face shape form the basis and ideals for evaluating and modifying all other face shapes.
    a. oblong
    b. heart-shaped
    c. round
    d. oval

    ____

32. Color acts as an illusion and helps to create lines of _____.

    a. direction   **c.** light

    b. attention   **d.** subtlety   ____

33. Depending on _____, color can accent or de-emphasize a particular part of a style or client feature.

    a. placement   **c.** hair length

    b. level   **d.** hair texture   ____

34. In hair design, the stylist follows five key strategies for successful end results including having a vision, following a plan, working at the plan, trying again and again, and _____.

    a. organizing your thoughts

    b. developing a strong foundation

    c. taking calculated risks

    d. looking to the past   ____

35. The _____ face shape features a long, narrow face with hollow cheeks.

    a. square   **c.** oblong

    b. triangular   **d.** round   ____

15 SCALP CARE, SHAMPOOING, & CONDITIONING

1. What is the primary purpose of a shampoo service?
   a. To recommend additional services
   b. To cleanse the hair and scalp
   c. To diagnose scalp diseases
   d. To analyze the scalp   ____

2. Which of the following is classified as a universal solvent?
   a. Salt   c. Lye
   b. Soap   d. Water   ____

3. Before water enters public water pipelines, small amounts
   of chlorine are added to water to _____.
   a. kill bacteria   c. soften the water
   b. add minerals   d. harden the water   ____

4. The ingredients on shampoo labels are listed in what order?
   a. In descending order from largest to smallest
   b. From smallest to largest percentage
   c. By similarity of ingredients
   d. Alphabetical order   ____

5. A pH-balanced shampoo has a pH in the range
   of _____.
   a. 3.0 to 3.0   c. 6.0 to 7.0
   b. 4.5 to 5.5   d. 7.5 to 8.5   ____

6. Which of the following are substances that absorb moisture
   or promote the retention of moisture?
   a. Proteins   c. Humectants
   b. Silicones   d. Preservatives   ____

7. A _____ is designed to penetrate the cortex
   and reinforce the hair shaft from within to temporarily
   reconstruct the hair.
   a. cleansing conditioner   c. leave-in conditioner
   b. scalp conditioner   d. protein conditioner   ____

8. Which of the following is used after a scalp treatment and before styling to remove oil accumulation from the scalp?
   a. Medicated scalp lotion
   b. Scalp astringent lotion
   c. Scalp conditioner
   d. Leave-in conditioner ____

9. Brushing of the hair should be avoided prior to _____.
   a. chemical services
   b. shampoo services
   c. styling services
   d. conditioning services ____

10. The most highly recommended hairbrushes are those made from _____.
    a. nylon bristles
    b. plastic bristles
    c. natural bristles
    d. metal bristles ____

11. As a safety feature for the client, during a shampoo you should monitor the water temperature by _____.
    a. waiting for the client to direct you to make it warmer or cooler
    b. keeping fingers under the spray
    c. using the nozzle to spray your palms periodically
    d. periodically dipping your elbow into the water ____

12. A dry hair and scalp treatment, used when there is a deficiency of natural oil on the hair or scalp, should contain _____.
    a. mineral oil base products
    b. sulfonated oil base products
    c. strong soap preparations
    d. moisturizing and emollient ingredients ____

13. A method of manipulating the scalp by rubbing, tapping, kneading, or _____ it with the hands is known as massage.
    a. stretching
    b. stroking
    c. softening
    d. scratching ____

14. Excessive oiliness is caused by _____.
    a. clogged pores
    b. a fungus called malassezia
    c. overactive sebaceous glands
    d. inactive sebaceous glands ____

15. When working a shampoo into a lather, you should use _____.
    a. the cushions of fingertips.   **c.** your palms
    b. your nails   **d.** the sides of your fingers   ____

16. The main difference between a relaxation massage and a treatment massage is _____.
    a. the duration of the massage
    b. the type of drape used
    c. your finger movements
    d. the products you use   ____

17. A shampoo should be selected according to _____.
    a. the condition of the client's hair and scalp
    b. the amount of money the client is willing to pay
    c. the type of shampoo you have the most of in stock
    d. the type of service planned after the shampoo   ____

18. Color-enhancing shampoos are used to _____.
    a. dull the color of the hair
    b. add a great deal of color to the hair
    c. add brassiness to the hair
    d. eliminate unwanted color tones   ____

19. Treatment or repair conditioners are deep, penetrating conditioners that restore _____ and moisture to the hair.
    a. keratin   **c.** nourishment
    b. protein   **d.** silicone   ____

20. A spray-on thermal protector is applied to the hair prior to any thermal service to protect the hair from the harmful effects of _____.
    a. cutting   **c.** conditioning
    b. shampooing   **d.** blowdrying   ____

21. For a client with _____ hair, it is recommended that you use a gentle cleansing shampoo and a light leave-in conditioner.
    a. dry and damaged, fine   **c.** curly, medium
    b. fine, straight   **d.** curly, coarse   ____

22. Appropriate products for coarse, dry and damaged hair include _____.
    a. volumizing shampoo
    b. finishing rinse
    c. spray-on thermal protector treatments
    d. deep-conditioning treatments and hair masks ____

23. Part One of the Three-Part Procedure for hair-care services includes _____.
    a. helping your client through the scheduling and payment process
    b. performing the actual service the client has requested
    c. cleaning and disinfecting your tools, implements, and materials
    d. advising the client and promoting products ____

24. What is the correct way to rinse your implements after cleaning them?
    a. Hold them under warm running water.
    b. Hold them under cold running water.
    c. Dip them into a tub of warm water.
    d. Dip them directly into disinfectant. ____

25. During the post-service procedure, it is important to determine if the client is satisfied, advise the client about proper at-home maintenance, and _____.
    a. discuss upcoming social events
    b. discuss retail product recommendations
    c. explain pending price increases
    d. review your service portfolio ____

26. Rainwater or chemically treated water that contains only a small amount of minerals is called _____.
    a. soft water   c. deionized water
    b. hard water   d. sparkling water ____

27. Water that contains minerals that reduce the ability of soap or shampoo to lather is called _____.
    a. soft water   c. deionized water
    b. hard water   d. distilled water ____

28. When offering a scalp massage, use slow, deliberate motions and _____.
    a. a firm touch   c. hard strokes
    b. mechanical movements d. a soft touch ____

29. A shampoo that contains special ingredients that are very effective in reducing dandruff or relieving other scalp conditions is called _____ shampoo.
  a. balancing
  b. clarifying
  c. medicated
  d. nonstripping

_____

30. Shampoo designed to make the hair appear smooth and shiny and to improve the manageability of the hair is called _____ shampoo.
  a. clarifying
  b. conditioning
  c. balancing
  d. medicated

_____

31. Shampoo containing an active chelating agent that binds to metals and removes them from the hair is called _____ shampoo.
  a. clarifying
  b. chelating
  c. conditioning
  d. balancing

_____

32. Shampoo designed to wash away excess oiliness, while preventing the hair from drying out, is called _____ shampoo
  a. balancing
  b. clarifying
  c. conditioning
  d. medicated

_____

33. Shampoo that cleanses the hair without the use of soap and water is _____ shampoo.
  a. humectant
  b. soft
  c. dry
  d. astringent

_____

34. The _____ end of a surfactant molecule is water-attracting.
  a. lipophilic
  b. humectant
  c. hydrophilic
  d. astringent

_____

35. Before the draping service, make sure that proper infection control practices are used and that each cape has been _____ prior to use.
  a. thoroughly rinsed and dried
  b. unfolded and aired out
  c. rendered wrinkle free
  d. laundered in a disinfecting solution

_____

36. A conditioner is a special chemical agent applied to the hair to deposit protein or moisturizer to help restore the hair's strength, _____, give hair body, and to protect hair against possible breakage.
    a. dehydrate
    b. infuse moisture
    c. remove oil
    d. repair hair
    ____

37. Shampoos formulated with little to no alkaline soap base are known as _____.
    a. sulfate-free
    b. color-enhancing
    c. neutralizing
    d. strengthening
    ____

38. The more alkaline the shampoo, the _____ it is.
    a. milder and more neutral
    b. stronger and more helpful
    c. stronger and harsher
    d. milder and sudsy
    ____

39. Prior to any service, analyze the client's hair and scalp and check for which of the following conditions?
    a. Hair color
    b. Thinning of the hair
    c. Percentage of gray
    d. Density of the hair
    ____

40. The _____ end of a surfactant molecule is oil-attracting.
    a. humectant
    b. hydrophilic
    c. astringent
    d. lipophilic
    ____

16 HAIRCUTTING

1. The reference point that signals a change in head shape from flat to round or vice versa is the _____.
   - **a.** crown area
   - **b.** occipital corner
   - **c.** four corners
   - **d.** parietal ridge
   ____

2. The straight lines used to build weight and create one-length and low-elevation haircuts are _____.
   - **a.** parallel lines
   - **b.** horizontal lines
   - **c.** weight lines
   - **d.** diagonal lines
   ____

3. The straight lines used to remove weight to create graduated or layered haircuts are _____.
   - **a.** cutting lines
   - **b.** diagonal lines
   - **c.** vertical lines
   - **d.** horizontal lines
   ____

4. For control during haircutting, the hair is parted into working areas called _____.
   - **a.** foundations
   - **b.** lines
   - **c.** parts
   - **d.** sections
   ____

5. The angle at which the fingers are held when cutting the line that creates the end shape is the _____.
   - **a.** elevation
   - **b.** guideline
   - **c.** cutting line
   - **d.** perimeter line
   ____

6. Which guideline is used when creating layers or a graduated haircut?
   - **a.** Traveling guideline
   - **b.** Outer guideline
   - **c.** Stationary guideline
   - **d.** Shape guideline
   ____

7. The technique of combing the hair away from its natural falling position, rather than straight out from the head, is called _____.
   - **a.** subsectioning
   - **b.** overdirection
   - **c.** traveling guidelines
   - **d.** undercutting
   ____

8. For a client with a long face, the stylist would recommend a style that adds _____.
   a. volume and height on top
   b. fullness on the sides
   c. weight to the chin and front
   d. fullness in length _____

9. A stylist will need to use less elevation on curly hair than on straighter textures, or leave the hair a bit longer because of _____.
   a. elasticity
   b. growth
   c. porosity
   d. shrinkage _____

10. The direction in which the hair grows from the scalp, also referred to as natural fall or natural falling position, is the _____.
    a. outermost perimeter
    b. fringe area
    c. parallel section
    d. growth pattern _____

11. Which type of comb is used for close tapers on the nape and sides when using the scissors-over-comb technique?
    a. Wide-toothed comb
    b. Barber comb
    c. Tail comb
    d. Styling comb _____

12. The technique used to free up the cutting hand to cut a subsection is called _____.
    a. moving the shears
    b. removing the comb
    c. transferring the comb
    d. working the shears _____

13. The term used to describe the amount of pressure applied when combing and holding a subsection is _____.
    a. tension
    b. sectioning
    c. elevation
    d. angle _____

14. When cutting hair, a general rule of thumb is to stand or sit _____.
    a. directly behind the area you are cutting
    b. directly in front of the area you are cutting
    c. to the right of the area you are cutting
    d. to the left of the area you are cutting _____

15. When cutting a(n) _____, it is customary to use a horizontal cutting line and cut below your fingers or on the insides of your knuckles.
    a. uniform or an increasing layered haircut
    b. high level layered effect or a bi-level cut
    c. shorter layer haircut or a shag effect
    d. blunt haircut or a heavier graduated haircut   ____

16. The visual line in a haircut, where the ends of the hair hang together, is the _____.
    a. guideline   c. graduated line
    b. weight line   d. stationary line   ____

17. Parting a haircut in the opposite way it was cut, at the same elevation, to check for precision of line and shape is called _____.
    a. cross-checking   c. mirror elevation
    b. consistent tension   d. blunt cutting   ____

18. If using the wide teeth of the comb while cutting a blunt haircut, always comb the section first with the fine teeth, then _____.
    a. change the position of the comb so it is at an angle
    b. switch the comb to the alternate hand and comb with the fine teeth
    c. turn the comb around and re-comb with the wide teeth
    d. turn the comb on its side and comb again   ____

19. It is important to work with _____, where and how hair is moved over the head, when locating the bang area.
    a. the head form   c. the fringe
    b. the natural distribution   d. the weight line   ____

20. A method of cutting or layering the hair in which the fingers and shears glide along the edge of the hair to remove length is _____.
    a. angle cutting   c. blunt cutting
    b. razor cutting   d. slide cutting   ____

21. The process of removing excess bulk without shortening hair length is known as _____.
    a. blunt cutting   c. texturizing
    b. angle cutting   d. compensating   ____

22. The process of thinning the hair to graduated lengths using a sliding movement of the shears with the blades kept partially open is called _____.
    a. slithering
    b. notching
    c. point cutting
    d. angle cutting ____

23. When performing the slicing technique to remove weight or on the surface of the haircut, it is best to work on _____.
    a. damp hair
    b. soapy hair
    c. wet hair
    d. dry hair ____

24. When using the clipper-over-comb technique, the amount of hair that is removed is determined by the _____.
    a. apex of the head
    b. angle of the comb
    c. size of the section
    d. type of clipper used ____

25. If the blade tension on your shears is too tight, it will cause the shears to bind and cause unnecessary wear and _____.
    a. user fatigue
    b. the adjustment knob to loosen
    c. the hair to fold
    d. debris to accumulate ____

26. The ability to duplicate an existing haircut or create a new haircut from a photo will build a stronger professional relationship between the stylist and _____.
    a. vendors
    b. manager
    c. clients
    d. fellow stylists ____

27. Elevation creates _____.
    a. graduation and layers
    b. cutting lines
    c. casts and crowns
    d. shrinkage ____

28. A guideline located at the outer line of the cut is known as the _____.
    a. parameter
    b. interior
    c. cutting line
    d. perimeter ____

29. Shears should be sharpened _____.
    a. after every service
    b. only as needed
    c. every three months
    d. every six months ____

30. You should use _____ tension on straight hair when you want precise lines.
   a. minimal
   c. moderate
   b. maximum
   d. zero ____

31. Using a razor on _____ hair will weaken the cuticle and cause frizzing.
   a. straight
   c. blond
   b. fine
   d. curly ____

32. A great haircut always begins with a _____.
   a. great consultation
   c. scalp massage
   b. good shampoo
   d. styling book ____

33. The client's hair should be _____ before the consultation.
   a. uncleansed and styled
   c. cleansed and styled
   b. uncleansed and unstyled
   d. cleansed and unstyled ____

34. A quick way to analyze a face shape is to determine if it is _____.
   a. long or short
   c. wide or long
   b. wide or narrow
   d. narrow or long ____

35. Hair texture is based on the _____ of each hair strand.
   a. length
   c. color
   b. thickness
   d. circumference ____

36. Hair density is the number of individual hair strands on _____ of scalp.
   a. 1/4 square inch
   c. 1/2 square inch
   b. 1/3 square inch
   d. 1 square inch ____

37. Clippers _____.
   a. are mainly used when creating long haircuts
   b. must never be used without a guard
   c. are mainly used to remove bulk from the hair
   d. may be used with cutting guards of various lengths ____

38. Cast shears are usually _____ than forged shears.
   a. less expensive to purchase
   b. more expensive to produce
   c. easier to bend back into shape
   d. denser ____

39. The _____ on a pair of shears allows you to have more control over the shear.
    a. cutting edge
    b. thumb hole
    c. finger tang
    d. pivot and the adjustment area   ____

40. Your shears should be cleaned and lubricated _____.
    a. after every client   c. once a week
    b. at the end of the day   d. as needed   ____

41. Before purchasing a pair of shears, ensure that the company has a person who is certified to _____ them in your area.
    a. clean   c. polish
    b. lubricate   d. sharpen   ____

42. Knowing how to hold your tools properly will help you avoid muscle strain in your _____.
    a. legs   c. chest
    b. shoulders   d. arms   ____

43. When palming the shears, hold the comb between your _____ fingers.
    a. thumb, index, and middle
    b. index, middle, and ring
    c. middle, ring, and pinky
    d. thumb, middle, and pinky   ____

44. To achieve constant, even results in a haircut, it is important to use _____ tension.
    a. minimum   c. maximum
    b. moderate   d. consistent   ____

45. Heavier graduated haircuts work well on hair that tends to _____ when dry.
    a. contract   c. become curlier
    b. expand   d. become shinier   ____

46. Which of these statements about cutting hair with a razor is true?
    a. A shear cut gives a softer appearance than a razor cut.
    b. A razor gives a softer effect on the ends of the hair than shears.
    c. Shears have much finer blades than razors.
    d. When working with a razor, the line is blunt.   ____

47. Texturizing *cannot* be done with _____.
     a. cutting shears   c. a razor
     b. thinning sheers   d. clippers   ____

48. When using clippers, you should always
     work _____ the natural growth patterns,
     especially in the nape.
     a. with
     b. against
     c. across
     d. alternately with and against   ____

49. When trimming a male client's facial hair, it is recommended
     that you check _____ and ask if he would like you
     to remove any excess hair.
     a. his ears only
     b. his eyebrows only
     c. his ears and eyebrows
     d. his chest   ____

50. Tho torm _____ refers to the shape of the head.
     a. head form   c. head guide
     b. skull form   d. guideline   ____

51. Places on the head that mark where the surface of the head
     changes are known as _____.
     a. four corners   c. reference points
     b. angles   d. perimeters   ____

52. The widest area of the head is the _____.
     a. occipital bone   c. nape
     b. parietal ridge   d. apex   ____

53. The bone that protrudes at the base of the skull is
     the _____.
     a. parietal ridge   c. occipital bone
     b. orbital bone   d. nape   ____

54. The highest point on the top of the head is
     the _____.
     a. apex   c. plateau
     b. peak   d. nape   ____

55. The area at the back part of the neck is the _____.
     a. bevel   c. notch
     b. cast   d. nape   ____

56. The triangular section that begins at the apex and ends at the front corners is the _____.
   a. back area
   b. bang area
   c. bevel area
   d. crown area
   _____

57. A _____ is a thin, continuous mark used as a guide.
   a. line
   b. head form
   c. layer
   d. part
   _____

58. Lines parallel from the floor and relative to the horizon are _____ lines.
   a. vertical
   b. horizontal
   c. diagonal
   d. straight
   _____

59. The space between two lines or surfaces that intersect at a given point is _____.
   a. an angle
   b. an apex
   c. a bevel
   d. an intersection
   _____

60. Lines perpendicular to the horizon are _____ lines.
   a. horizontal
   b. straight
   c. diagonal
   d. vertical
   _____

61. Lines that have a slanting or sloping direction are _____ lines.
   a. straight
   b. horizontal
   c. vertical
   d. diagonal
   _____

62. The line dividing the hair at the scalp is a _____.
   a. part
   b. bevel
   c. section
   d. graduation
   _____

63. When creating uniform layers, the hair is elevated to _____ degrees from the scalp and cut at the same length.
   a. 180
   b. 90
   c. 60
   d. 45
   _____

64. What type of shear blade edge gives the smoothest cut and has the sharpest edge possible?
   a. A full concave edge
   b. A partial concave edge
   c. A full convex edge
   d. A partial beveled edge
   _____

65. When purchasing shears, consider purchasing a shear that comes with a _____ system since you will be working with the shears almost constantly.
   a. form-fitting
   b. self-adjusting
   c. self-beveling
   d. finger-fitting
   ____

66. Which type of texture shears is the best for adding increased blending?
   a. Blending shear
   b. Texturizing shear
   c. Chunking shear
   d. Thinning shear
   ____

67. _____ is the key to avoiding long-term repetitive motion injuries and other musculoskeletal disorders.
   a. Prevention
   b. Relaxation
   c. Exercise
   d. Practice
   ____

68. Which hand position is used most often when cutting uniform or increasing layers?
   a. Cutting below the fingers
   b. Cutting palm-to-palm
   c. Cutting over your fingers
   d. Cutting across the palm
   ____

69. Which haircut is cut at a 90-degree elevation and then overdirected to maintain length and weight at the perimeter?
   a. The layered haircut
   b. The long-layered haircut
   c. The blunt haircut
   d. The bob haircut
   ____

70. Always make consistent and _____ partings, which will give an even amount of hair to each subsection and produce more precise results.
   a. thin
   b. short
   c. thick
   d. clean
   ____

71. When cutting a layered haircut on a client with hair past the shoulder blades, which technique is used to connect the top sections to the lengths?
   a. Texturizing
   b. Scissor-over-comb
   c. Slide cutting
   d. Clipper cutting
   ____

72. Which cutting tool should generally be avoided when cutting curly hair?
   a. Razor
   b. Clipper
   c. Shear
   d. Texturizing shear
   ____

73. When using the scissor-over-comb technique, how is the haircut cross-checked?
   a. By working across the area horizontally
   b. By working across the area vertically
   c. By working across the area diagonally
   d. By cutting across the wide teeth of the comb ____

74. Which haircut represents cutting the hair very short and close to the hairline and then gradually getting longer as you move up the head?
   a. A blunt cut   c. A fade
   b. A layer cut   d. A taper ____

75. What is the process called when the hair contracts or lifts through the action of moisture loss/drying?
   a. Reduction   c. Contraction
   b. Shrinkage   d. Parting ____

CHAPTER 17 HAIRSTYLING

1. The first step in the hairstyling process is always
   the _____.
   a. cool water shampoo
   c. client consultation
   b. draping procedure
   d. conditioning treatment _____

2. The process of shaping and directing the hair into an S
   pattern through the use of the fingers, combs, and finger-
   waving lotion is called _____.
   a. hairstyling
   c. ridge curls
   b. finger waving
   d. roller setting _____

3. In creating horizontal finger waves, the waves are
   placed _____.
   a. up and down the head
   b. on the heavy side of the head
   c. down and parallel
   d. sideways and parallel around the head _____

4. The stationary foundation of a pin curl is
   the _____.
   a. base
   c. section
   b. curl
   d. stem _____

5. Pin curls that produce tight, firm, long-lasting curls and
   allow for minimum mobility are known as _____.
   a. off-base pin curls
   c. on-base pin curls
   b. half-stem pin curls
   d. no-stem pin curls _____

6. Pin curls formed in a shaping should begin at
   the _____.
   a. open end
   c. odd side
   b. closed side
   d. shaping side _____

7. The most commonly shaped pin curl bases are rectangular,
   triangular, square, or _____.
   a. s-shaped
   c. no-base
   b. arc based
   d. circular _____

8. Pin curls sliced from a shaping and formed without lifting the hair from the head are referred to as _____.

    a. stem curls   **c.** carved curls

    b. design curls   **d.** ridge curls   ____

9. The panel of hair on which a roller is placed is the _____.

    a. stem   **c.** base

    b. section   **d.** subsection   ____

10. Hair between the scalp and the first turn of the roller is the _____.

    a. curl   **c.** arc

    b. base   **d.** stem   ____

11. The point where curls of opposite directions meet, forming a recessed area is called the _____.

    a. indentation   **c.** divot

    b. convex   **d.** wave   ____

12. To smooth hair that is backcombed, hold the teeth of a comb or the bristles of a brush at a _____ pointing away from you, and lightly move the comb over the surface of the hair.

    a. 15-degree angle   **c.** 90-degree angle

    b. 45-degree angle   **d.** 0-degree angle   ____

13. Which type of styling product is also known as mousse?

    a. Texturizer   **c.** Styling gel

    b. Holding spray   **d.** Foam   ____

14. A benefit of using _____ is that they offer firmer, longer hold for fine hair with the least amount of heaviness.

    a. heavy gels with weight   **c.** texturizers

    b. finishing sprays   **d.** pomades   ____

15. Which of these styling aids is applied to damp hair (ranging from wavy to extremely curly) and then blown dry to create a smooth, straight look that provides the most hold in dry outdoor conditions?

    a. Foam   **c.** Spray gel

    b. Straightening gel   **d.** Mousse   ____

16. One way to remove dirt, oils, and product residue from a thermal iron is to use a dampened towel or rag and wipe down the barrel of the iron with a soapy solution containing a few drops of _____.
    a. styling gel
    b. peroxide
    c. ammonia
    d. bleach
    _____

17. Which of the following is a technique used to temporarily straighten extremely curly or resistant hair until the hair is shampooed?
    a. Hair pressing
    b. Blowdrying
    c. Thermal curling
    d. Deep cleansing
    _____

18. Applying a thermal pressing comb twice on each side of the hair to remove curl is a _____.
    a. hard press
    b. soft press
    c. thermal press
    d. medium press
    _____

19. A tight scalp can be made more flexible with hair brushing and the systematic use of _____.
    a. conditioning masks
    b. scalp massage
    c. conditioning shampoos
    d. roller sets
    _____

20. When executing an updo, stand back and away from your work to make sure the _____ is right, and use the mirror and look at every angle.
    a. height
    b. balance
    c. volume
    d. effect
    _____

21. After heating the iron to the desired temperature, test it on _____.
    a. the client's hair
    b. your own hair
    c. a piece of tissue paper
    d. your finger
    _____

22. When using rollers, one and a half turns will create _____.
    a. a wave
    b. curls
    c. an indentation
    d. a C-shape curl
    _____

23. Hot rollers are to be used only on _____.
    a. wet hair
    b. damp hair
    c. dry hair
    d. curly hair
    _____

24. The French Pleat is an elegant, sleek look that can be worn for any occasion, but clients are most likely to request it for _____.
    a. a relaxing summer style
    b. a warming winter style
    c. casual activities
    d. a formal function ____

25. How long do Velcro™ rollers need to stay in the hair?
    a. 5 to 10 minutes
    b. 10 to 15 minutes
    c. 15 to 20 minutes
    d. 20 to 30 minutes ____

26. Hair wrapping can be done _____.
    a. only on wet hair
    b. only on dry hair
    c. only on damp hair
    d. on wet or dry hair ____

27. The technique of drying and styling damp hair in one operation is called _____.
    a. shaping
    b. blowdry styling
    c. unistyling
    d. hair wrapping ____

28. The blowdryer's nozzle attachment, or _____, is a directional feature that creates a concentrated stream of air.
    a. volumizer
    b. stem
    c. diffuser
    d. concentrator ____

29. Thermal waving and curling is also known as _____.
    a. thio waving
    b. straight waving
    c. Marcel waving
    d. shell waving ____

30. Nonelectric thermal irons are favored by many stylists who cater to clients with _____ hair.
    a. straight
    b. wavy
    c. curly
    d. excessively curly ____

31. What is the best way to practice manipulative techniques with thermal irons?
    a. Rolling the cold iron in your hand, first forward and then backward
    b. Rolling the cold iron in your hand, first backward and then forward
    c. Rolling the warmed iron in your hand, first forward and then backward
    d. Rolling the warmed iron in your hand, first backward and then forward ____

32. A modern thermal iron and _____ are all you need to give your client curls.
   a. a nylon brush   **c.** a hard rubber comb
   b. a clipper   **d.** a wide tooth comb   ____

33. End curls can be used to give a finished appearance to _____.
   a. the cortex   **c.** hair root
   b. hair ends   **d.** the style balance   ____

34. Full-base curls sit in the center of their base and provide _____ with full volume.
   a. a weak curl   **c.** little movement
   b. a strong curl   **d.** a medium curl   ____

35. Who can diagnose scalp skin disease?
   a. A dermatologist   **c.** A podiatrist
   b. A cosmetologist   **d.** A pulmonologist   ____

36. Coarse hair requires _____ to press than medium or fine hair.
   a. more heat and pressure   **c.** little pressure
   b. less heat and pressure   **d.** less tension   ____

37. When tempering a new pressing comb, you should _____.
   a. heat the comb until it is extremely hot
   b. coat the comb in olive oil
   c. cool the comb in a freezer
   d. rinse the comb under cold running water to remove the oil   ____

38. Which of the following is usually recommended at the side front hairline for a smooth, upswept effect?
   a. Barrel curls   **c.** Cascade curls
   b. Rectangular base pin curls   **d.** Square base pin curls   ____

39. Which type of curl is usually recommended along the front or facial hairline to prevent breaks or splits in the finished hairstyle?
   a. Ridge curl
   b. Cascade curl
   c. Triangular base pin curl
   d. Rectangular base curl   ____

40. Which type of curl is suitable for curly hairstyles without much volume and lift, can be used on any part of the head, and will comb out with lasting results?
    a. Ridge curl
    b. Barrel curl
    c. Rectangular base curl
    d. Square base pin curl ____

41. Where are skip waves usually found?
    a. The side of the head
    b. The back of the head
    c. The top of the head
    d. The forehead ____

42. Pin curls placed immediately behind or below a ridge to form a wave are called _____.
    a. triangular base curls
    b. cascade curls
    c. barrel curls
    d. ridge curls ____

43. Which type of curls are also known as stand-up curls?
    a. Rectangular base curls
    b. Cascade curls
    c. Ridge curls
    d. Triangular base pin curls ____

44. Which type of curls have large center openings and are fastened to the head in a standing position on a rectangular base?
    a. Cascade curls
    b. Ridge curls
    c. Barrel curls
    d. Square base pin curls ____

45. Which roller position is recommended for full volume?
    a. On base
    b. Off base
    c. Half base
    d. Dual base ____

46. Which roller position is recommended for the least volume?
    a. On base
    b. Off base
    c. Half base
    d. Dual base ____

47. Which of these is used to build a soft cushion or to mesh two or more curl patterns together for a uniform and smooth comb out?
    a. Sidecombing
    b. Sidebrushing
    c. Backcombing
    d. Backbrushing ____

48. Which of these involves combing small sections of hair from the ends toward the scalp, causing shorter hair to mat at the scalp and form a cushion or base?
    a. Sidecombing
    b. Sidebrushing
    c. Backcombing
    d. Backbrushing ____

49. A _____ is a half-round, rubber-based brush.
   a. vent brush
   b. grooming brush
   c. classic styling brush
   d. teasing brush   ____

50. A _____ is generally an oval brush with a mixture of boar and nylon bristles.
   a. vent brush
   b. grooming brush
   c. classic styling brush
   d. teasing brush   ____

51. A _____ is a thin, nylon styling brush that has a tail for sectioning, along with a narrow row of bristles.
   a. vent brush
   b. grooming brush
   c. classic styling brush
   d. teasing brush   ____

52. A _____ is a brush used to speed up the blowdrying process.
   a. vent brush
   b. grooming brush
   c. classic styling brush
   d. teasing brush   ____

53. Sleek bobs with finger waves and pin curls were popular during the _____.
   a. 1920s and 1930s
   b. 1940s and 1950s
   c. 1960s and 1970s
   d. 1980s and 1990s   ____

54. Arc base pin curls are also known as _____.
   a. S-curls
   b. V-curls
   c. half-moon curls
   d. full-moon curls   ____

55. Which part of a roller curl is also known as the circle?
   a. The base
   b. The curl
   c. The stem
   d. The paddle   ____

56. How many times do you turn the roller to create a C-shape curl?
   a. One
   b. One and a half
   c. Two
   d. Two and a half   ____

57. Velcro™ rollers can be used _____.
   a. only on wet hair
   b. only on dry hair
   c. only on damp hair
   d. on wet, dry, or damp hair ____

58. A section of hair that is molded in a circular movement in preparation for the formation of curls is called a _____.
   a. half moon
   b. molding
   c. circle
   d. shaping   ____

59. When you use a comb with teeth spaced closely together, it _____.

    a. removes definition from the surface
    b. lifts hair away from the surface
    c. removes definition from the curl
    d. creates a rough surface   ____

60. Which type of styling product is also known as wax?

    a. Pomade   **c.** Finishing spray
    b. Silicone   **d.** Volumizer   ____

61. In thermal curling, the hair is held at a 70-degree angle for _____.

    a. half-base curls   **c.** full-base curls
    b. off-base curls   **d.** volume-base curls   ____

62. With a stove-heated pressing comb, remove the carbon by rubbing the outside surface and between the teeth with fine sandpaper or _____.

    a. a scouring pad   **c.** wet sponge
    b. a microfiber cloth   **d.** a fine steel-wool pad   ____

63. What is recommended to help repair and moisturize the hair and scalp that has been pressed?

    a. Frequent shampooing
    b. Using perfumed pressing oil
    c. A conditioning treatment mask
    d. Adding pomade after pressing   ____

64. What is a special consideration when pressing coarse hair?

    a. Apply enough pressure so that hair remains straightened.
    b. Avoid using a hot pressing comb.
    c. Apply 4 percent gentian violet jelly to the hair strands.
    d. Apply only moderate pressure for a brief amount of time.   ____

65. The foundation technique used for the classic bun or the chignon is the _____.

    a. fishtail braid   **c.** pleat
    b. ponytail   **d.** twist   ____

CHAPTER 18 BRAIDING & BRAID EXTENSIONS

1. Hair care that uses no chemicals or dyes and does not alter the natural curl or coil pattern of the hair, is known as _____.
   a. chemical-free hairstyling
   b. synthetic hairstyling
   c. natural hairstyling
   d. curl-free hair care   ____

2. Which of the following braid style or length is recommended for a client with a square face?
   a. A style with more width at the sides
   b. A style with height
   c. Using bangs or sweep braids across the forehead
   d. Framing the face with longer braids   ____

3. The _____ face is a too-long oval and requires a style with more width at the sides.
   a. pear-shaped
   b. elongated
   c. oval
   d. heart-shaped   ____

4. Which brush is recommended for stimulating the scalp and removing dirt and lint from locks?
   a. Vent brush
   b. Boar-bristle brush
   c. Nylon-bristle brush
   d. Square paddle brush   ____

5. Which of the following is a characteristic of Kanekalon?
   a. It closely mimics human hair.
   b. It is not very durable.
   c. It is not heat-resistant.
   d. It is prone to tangling.   ____

6. When curly hair is braided wet, it _____ as it dries.
   a. stretches significantly
   b. remains unchanged
   c. expands slightly
   d. shrinks and recoils   ____

7. Which type of braid is a three-strand braid that is created with an underhand technique?
   a. French
   b. Inverted
   c. Visible
   d. Invisible   ____

8. Single braids can move _____.
   a. in any direction
   b. from side to side
   c. up and down
   d. diagonally
   _____

9. Extensions for single braids are integrated into natural hair using the _____.
   a. two-strand overhand technique
   b. three-strand underhand technique
   c. individual braid technique
   d. medium to large techniques
   _____

10. Which of the following is not a basic method of locking?
    a. The coil comb technique
    b. Braids or extensions
    c. The palm roll
    d. Brotherlocks
    _____

11. In some African tribes, different styles of braiding indicated _____.
    a. a person's social status
    b. the family to which a person belonged
    c. whether the person had children
    d. whether the person was married
    _____

12. What is the most important feature of the wide-tooth comb?
    a. The length of the teeth
    b. The distance between the teeth
    c. The material from which the comb is made
    d. The sharpness of the teeth
    _____

13. Most human hair used for hair extensions is imported from which part of the world?
    a. South America
    b. Asia
    c. Eastern Europe
    d. South Africa
    _____

14. Blowdrying dries the hair quickly, softens the hair in the process, and makes _____.
    a. the wave pattern tighter
    b. the hair-shaft shorter
    c. it more manageable for combing and sectioning
    d. pick up and manipulation slightly more difficult
    _____

15. The fishtail braid is best done on _____.
    a. shoulder length, layered hair
    b. short, layered hair
    c. shoulder length or longer, non-layered hair
    d. short, non-layered hair
    _____

16. Braiders report that tree braids take about _____ hours.
    a. three   c. five
    b. four   d. six   ____

17. During which developmental phase of locks can a bulb be
    felt at the end of each lock?
    a. Sprouting stage   c. Pre-lock stage
    b. Growing stage   d. Maturation stage   ____

18. During which developmental phase of locks does the hair
    begin to regain length?
    a. Sprouting stage   c. Pre-lock stage
    b. Growing stage   d. Maturation stage   ____

19. During the first developmental phase of locks, the hair
    coil _____.
    a. is rough in texture   c. is straight and dull
    b. has a matte texture   d. has an open end   ____

20. Which of the following is a braid created with two strands
    that are twisted around each other?
    a. Fishtail braid   c. Rope braid
    b. Invisible braid   d. Single braid   ____

21. Which of the following are separate networks of curly,
    textured hair that have been intertwined and meshed
    together?
    a. French braids   c. Cornrows
    b. Locks   d. Canerows

22. A _____ is used to dry hair without disturbing the
    enhanced curl pattern and without dehydrating the hair.
    a. hood dryer   c. concentrator
    b. pick nozzle   d. diffuser   ____

23. The practice of overlapping two strands to form a candy
    cane effect is known as _____.
    a. twisting   c. plaiting
    b. weaving   d. inverting   ____

24. When performing a braiding service, which essential tool
    is used for creating shapes and finished looks, and for
    trimming bangs and excess extension material?
    a. Two-inch scissors   c. Five-inch scissors
    b. Three-inch scissors   d. Electric trimmers   ____

25. The term _____ refers to narrow rows of visible braids that lie close to the scalp and are created with a three-stand, on-the-scalp braiding technique.
    a. cornrows
    b. locks
    c. twists
    d. dreadlocks ____

26. Which of the following is a tool that separates the hair as it combs, making it an excellent detangling comb for wet curly hair?
    a. Finishing comb
    b. Double-tooth comb
    c. Tail comb
    d. Cutting comb ____

27. Which of these is a tool used for cutting small sections, and should only be used after the hair has been blown dry?
    a. Finishing comb
    b. Double-toothed comb
    c. Tail comb
    d. Cutting comb ____

28. A _____ is useful for lifting and separating textured hair.
    a. wide-toothed comb
    b. square paddle brush
    c. pick with rounded teeth
    d. vent brush ____

29. Which of the following is a free-hanging braid, with or without an extension, that can be executed using either an underhand or an overhand technique?
    a. Inverted braid
    b. Single braid
    c. Plait braid
    d. Fishtail braid ____

30. Which type of brush is good for releasing tangles, knots, and snarls in short, textured hair and long, straight hair?
    a. Square paddle brush
    b. Boar-bristle brush
    c. Vent brush
    d. Natural hairbrush ____

31. What is the benefit of mixing yak hair with human hair?
    a. It makes the hair easier to color.
    b. It eliminates the need to shampoo the hair.
    c. It helps to remove the manufactured shine.
    d. It makes the hair easier to style. ____

32. Which of the following braids is not created with three strands and an overhand technique?
    a. French braid
    b. Invisible braid
    c. Inverted braid
    d. Rope braid ____

33. The _____ method builds up the braid strand by strand with extension hair fibers.
   a. feed-in
   b. over-weave
   c. draw-down
   d. button-through
   ____

34. A finishing comb is usually _____ in length and works well on fine or straight hair.
   a. 3 to 4 inches
   b. 5 to 6 inches
   c. 6 to 8 inches
   d. 8 to 10 inches
   ____

35. The flat leather pad with very close, fine teeth that sandwiches human hair extensions is called a _____.
   a. book board
   b. drawing board
   c. flat iron
   d. leather clamp
   ____

36. During analysis of the client's hair and scalp for a braiding service, you will pay particular attention to the hair's type and texture, _____, scalp abrasions, and hair thinning or balding.
   a. hair length
   b. hair color
   c. curl configuration
   d. skin type
   ____

37. Another term for wave pattern is _____.
   a. coil configuration
   b. curl pattern
   c. curl configuration
   d. coil pattern
   ____

38. The traditional _____ is flat, natural, and contoured to the scalp.
   a. invisible braid
   b. cornrow
   c. visible braid
   d. dreadlock
   ____

39. When the hair is double-strand twisted or coil twisted and wrapped around itself to make a knot, it is called a _____.
   a. braid-out set
   c. glamour wave
   c. flat-twist
   d. Bantu knot
   ____

40. When small sections of natural hair are gelled and spiraled with the fingers or a comb to create individual formations of tight, cylindrical coils, it is known as _____.
   a. coil-out
   b. a spiral rod set
   c. comb twists
   d. glamour waves
   ____

CHAPTER *19* WIGS & HAIR ADDITIONS

1. The fastest way to determine whether a strand of hair is synthetic is to _____.
   a. burn it with a match
   b. contact the manufacturer
   c. cut it with scissors
   d. wet and blow dry it
   _____

2. Which of the following is a disadvantage of synthetic hair?
   a. Synthetic hair always looks unnatural.
   b. Synthetic hair is more expensive than human hair.
   c. Synthetic hair cannot be exposed to extreme heat.
   d. Synthetic hair is more prone to fading.
   _____

3. When cutting a wig, the general goal is to make the hair _____.
   a. fit more snugly
   b. more fashionable
   c. more comfortable
   d. look more realistic
   _____

4. When cutting a wig using free-form cutting, always work _____.
   a. away from the weight
   b. toward the weight
   o. away from the forehead
   d. toward the forehead
   _____

5. Which method of wig construction is the least expensive?
   a. Hand-tied
   b. Semi-hand-tied
   c. Machine-made
   d. Artificially sewn
   _____

6. When shampooing a wig, it is recommended that you avoid shampoos that have _____ base.
   a. a sulfur
   b. an oil
   c. a carbon
   d. a nitrogen
   _____

7. Synthetic hair colors used on wigs and hairpieces are standardized according to the _____ colors on the hair color ring used by wig and hairpiece manufacturers.
   a. 50
   b. 70
   c. 90
   d. 110
   _____

8. The _____ is a sewing stitch in which the thread is wound around the needle twice.
   a. double-lock stitch
   c. overcast stitch
   b. secure lock stitch
   d. loop stitch
   ____

9. The _____ involves attaching hair wefts or single strands with an adhesive.
   a. track method
   c. sewing method
   b. lockstitch method
   d. bonding method
   ____

10. The fusion-bonding method of attaching hair extensions requires that the bonding material be activated by _____.
    a. a liquid activator
    c. water
    b. a catalyst
    d. heat
    ____

11. Which of the following is an advantage of using a hair addition made of human hair?
    a. It has less durability.
    b. It has a more realistic appearance.
    c. It never frizzes or loses its curl in humid weather.
    d. The color will not fade or oxidize.
    ____

12. When using heat on human hair, always set the styling tool on _____.
    a. low
    c. high
    b. medium
    d. ultra high
    ____

13. Traditionally, brushes made with _____ bristles have been regarded as best for use on human hair.
    a. metal
    c. natural boar
    b. straw
    d. nylon
    ____

14. A hair wrap is secured to the client's own hair with _____.
    a. combs
    c. a bandana
    b. hairpins
    d. fast-drying adhesive
    ____

15. When sewing on an extension using the braid-and-sew attachment method, it is recommended that you avoid using a _____ needle.
    a. straight
    c. curved
    b. custom-designed
    d. sharp
    ____

16. When bonding, it is recommended that you work _____ away from the hairline to keep the wefts from showing.
    a. one half inch
    b. one inch
    c. one and one half inches
    d. two inches _____

17. To use a linking method of attachment, the natural hair should be at least how long?
    a. 3 inches   c. 6 inches
    b. 5 inches   d. 8 inches _____

18. A small wig used to cover the top and crown of the head is _____.
    a. a toupee   c. a cap wig
    b. an integration hairpiece   d. partial weft _____

19. A _____ is a long strip of hair with a threaded edge.
    a. bond   c. root
    b. block   d. weft _____

20. A hairpiece that has openings in the base, through which the client's own hair is pulled to blend with the hair of the hairpiece, is _____.
    a. a semi-hand-tied wig   c. a hair extension
    b. an integration hairpiece   d. a capless wig _____

21. The head-shaped form on which a wig is secured for fitting, coloring, and sometimes styling is known as a _____.
    a. mount   c. block
    b. brand   d. cap _____

22. A hair addition secured to the base of the client's natural hair in order to add length, volume, texture, or color is _____.
    a. a hair extension   c. a cap wig
    b. a toupee   d. an integration hairpiece _____

23. A _____ is made by inserting individual strands of hair into mesh foundations and knotting them with a needle.
    a. cap wig   c. hand-tied wig
    b. capless wig   d. machine-made wig _____

24. Hair that has been shed from the head and gathered from a hairbrush is known as _____.
    a. bonded hair   c. turned hair
    b. carved hair   d. fallen hair   ____

25. A _____ is an artificial covering for the head consisting of a network of interwoven hair.
    a. wig   c. cap
    b. weft   d. block   ____

26. A wig constructed with an elasticized, mesh-fiber base to which the hair is attached is called a _____.
    a. capless wig   c. Remi wig
    b. cap wig   d. fusion bond   ____

27. Hair in which the root end of every single strand is sewn into the base is called _____.
    a. bonded hair   c. turned hair
    b. carved hair   d. fallen hair   ____

28. Wigs, hairpieces, and extensions made of modacrylic are particularly _____.
    a. unrealistic in appearance
    b. strong and durable
    c. weak, but flexible
    d. susceptible to sun damage   ____

29. Indian hair is usually _____.
    a. extremely curly   c. tightly coiled
    b. straight   d. wavy   ____

30. Average sized wigs fit heads from _____.
    a. 21.5 to 22.5 inches c. 19 to 21.5 inches
    b. 22.5 to 24 inches   d. 23.5 to 24.5 inches ____

31. The simple, quick stitch that can be used to secure the entire length of a weft to a track is the _____.
    a. double-lock stitch   c. lock stitch
    b. blunt stitch   d. overcast stitch   ____

32. Which type of hair extension covers the entire top and back of the head and allows the client to have longer, fuller curls?
    a. An integration piece c. A capless wig
    b. Cascading curls   d. A wrap around ponytail ____

33. If the hair in a human hair wig is porous, what is the best choice of hair color?
    a. Permanent   **c.** Semipermanent
    b. Temporary   **d.** Hair mascara   ____

34. Which type of hair is an excellent base for adding color?
    a. Yak hair   **c.** Remi hair
    b. Indian hair   **d.** Chinese hair   ____

35. When styling a wig, what is the best test to gauge how realistic the wig looks?
    a. The wind test   **c.** The flexibility test
    b. The strength test   **d.** The moisture test   ____

20 CHEMICAL TEXTURE SERVICES

1. The chemical texture service that loosens overly curly hair or changes tightly curly or coiled hair into loose curls or waves is _____.
   a. curl softening
   b. curl re-forming
   c. alternate waving
   d. swelling compound ____

2. The layer of the hair that provides the strength and elasticity of human hair is the _____.
   a. medulla
   b. regular
   c. cortex
   d. arrector ____

3. The natural pH of hair is between _____.
   a. 4.0 and 5.0
   b. 4.5 and 5.5
   c. 6.0 and 7.0
   d. 7.0 and 8.0 ____

4. In permanent waving, the size of the curl is determined by the _____.
   a. position of the rod
   b. length of the hair
   c. wrapping of the rod
   d. size of the rod ____

5. The technique of wrapping hair at an angle of 90 degrees or perpendicular to its base section is _____.
   a. half off-base placement
   b. on-base placement
   c. off-base placement
   d. full-base placement ____

6. The two basic types of wrapping the hair around a perm rod are the spiral and _____.
   a. loop technique
   b. croquignole perm technique
   c. placement technique
   d. horizontal technique ____

7. A reduction reaction involves either the addition of hydrogen or the removal of _____.
   a. oxygen
   b. peroxide
   c. carbon
   d. nitrogen ____

8. Most cold waves have a pH between _____.
   a. 9.0 and 9.6   c. 8.0 and 9.0
   b. 10.0 and 10.8   d. 7.6 and 8.4   ____

9. The three separate components of acid waves are permanent waving solution, activator, and _____.
   a. conditioner   c. neutralizer
   b. stabilizer   d. shampoo   ____

10. An endothermic wave is activated by _____.
    a. an ammonia lotion   c. a sulfite source
    b. an outside heat source   d. a reducing agent   ____

11. Permanent wave solution should be rinsed from the hair for at least _____.
    a. 2 minutes   c. 15 minutes
    b. 10 minutes   d. 5 minutes   ____

12. The process of rearranging the structure of curly hair into a straighter or smoother form is _____.
    a. chemical hair relaxing   c. continuation
    b. chemical smoothing   d. neutralizing   ____

13. Thio relaxers usually have a pH above _____.
    a. 5   c. 9
    b. 10   d. 6   ____

14. Hydroxide ions left in the hair after a relaxer can be neutralized using a(n) _____.
    a. acid-balanced shampoo   c. thio neutralizer
    b. conditioning rinse   d. acid-free shampoo   ____

15. Which type of relaxer contains only one component and is used exactly as it is packaged with no mixing necessary?
    a. Thio relaxers
    b. Lye-based relaxers
    c. Metal hydroxide relaxers
    d. Acid-based relaxers   ____

16. Lithium hydroxide and potassium hydroxide relaxers are often advertised and sold as _____.
    a. conditioner relaxers
    b. no mix—no lye relaxers
    c. no mix—no chemical relaxers
    d. lye relaxers   ____

17. Which type of bonds are relatively weak physical side bonds that are the result of an attraction between negative and positive electrical charges?
    a. Disulfide bonds
    c. Salt bonds
    b. Polypeptide bonds
    d. Waving bonds _____

18. Which type of rod is also known as a circle rod?
    a. Loop rods
    c. Concave rods
    b. Soft bender rods
    d. Straight rods _____

19. For on-base placement, the hair is wrapped at _____ beyond perpendicular to its base section, and the rod is positioned on its base.
    a. 180 degrees
    c. 90 degrees
    b. 15 degrees
    d. 45 degrees _____

20. Which of these permanent waves process at room temperature?
    a. Acid-balanced waves
    c. Low-pH waves
    b. Exothermic waves
    d. True acid waves _____

21. Chemical solutions _____ the pH of the hair to an alkaline state.
    a. lower
    c. neutralize
    b. raise
    d. do not affect _____

22. When should you perform an elasticity test?
    a. Before perming the hair
    c. After perming the hair
    b. While perming the hair
    d. Never _____

23. Porous hair _____.
    a. is difficult to penetrate
    b. should never be permed
    c. could be damaged by a highly alkaline permanent waving solution
    d. could be damaged by a highly acidic permanent waving solution _____

24. GMTG, the primary reducing agent in most acid waves, has _____.
    a. no pH
    c. a high pH
    b. a neutral pH
    d. a low pH _____

25. True acid waves have a pH between _____.
    a. 2.0 and 3.0
    c. 5.5 and 8.0
    b. 4.5 and 7.0
    d. 6.0 and 9.0 _____

26. Ammonia-free waves _____.
   a. have a very strong odor
   b. are very acidic
   c. contain some ammonia
   d. have very little odor   ____

27. In permanent waving, most of the processing takes place within the first _____.
   a. 5 to 10 minutes   **c.** 20 to 30 minutes
   b. 10 to 20 minutes   **d.** 45 to 60 minutes   ____

28. One safety precaution of permanent waving is to _____.
   a. perm hair that has previously been treated with hydroxide relaxers
   b. perm excessively damaged hair
   c. examine the scalp before the perm service
   d. perform a test for metallic salts only if the client requests it   ____

29. With extremely curly hair, the twists are the _____ sections of the hair stands.
   a. thickest and strongest   **c.** thickest and weakest
   b. thinnest and weakest   **d.** thinnest and strongest ____

30. Relaxers are _____ and can literally melt or dissolve hair if used incorrectly.
   a. extremely alkaline   **c.** mildly alkaline
   b. extremely acidic   **d.** mildly acidic   ____

31. If the client's hair has been treated with a hydroxide relaxer, it means the hair _____.
   a. has disulfide bonds that are in the process of reforming
   b. has strong disulfide bonds
   c. is ideal for permanent waving
   d. will not hold a curl when applying a thio relaxer or thio permanent   ____

32. A _____ is a perm wrap in which one end paper is placed under and another is placed over the strand of hair being wrapped.
   a. double flat wrap   **b.** bookend wrap
   c. croquignole perm wrap   **d.** single flat wrap   ____

33. Which types of rods are usually about 12 inches (30.5 centimeters) long with a uniform diameter along the entire length of the rod?
   a. Straight rods   **c.** Soft bender rods
   b. Loop rods   **d.** Concave rods   ____

34. Thioglycolic acid _____.
   a. has no odor
   b. is a common reducing agent
   c. is dark in color
   d. has a pleasant scent   ____

35. The _____ is the innermost layer of the hair.
   a. cortex   **c.** medulla
   b. base   **d.** cuticle   ____

36. The partings and bases radiate throughout the panels to follow the curvature of the head in which type of wrap?
   a. Bricklay permanent wrap
   b. Double flat wrap
   c. Spiral perm wrap
   d. Curvature permanent wrap   ____

37. The chemical bonds that join amino acids together are called _____.
   a. hydrogen bonds   **c.** disulfide bonds
   b. peptide bonds   **d.** thio bonds   ____

38. A _____ is a type of perm wrap in which the hair is wrapped at an angle other than perpendicular to the length of the rod.
   a. spiral perm wrap
   b. straight set wrap
   c. basic permanent wrap
   d. bookend wrap   ____

39. Which of the following is a method of hair straightening that combines the use of a thio relaxer with flat ironing?
   a. Weave technique
   b. Japanese thermal straightening
   c. Thio neutralization
   d. No-base relaxing straightening   ____

40. Which type of relaxer requires the application of a protective base cream to the entire scalp prior to the application of the relaxer?

- **a.** Hydroxide relaxer
- **b.** No-base relaxer
- **c.** Thio relaxer
- **d.** Base relaxer

____

41. The middle layer of the hair is the _____.

- **a.** medulla
- **b.** cuticle
- **c.** cortex
- **d.** base

____

42. Which of these terms refers to the angle at which the rod is positioned on the head: horizontally, vertically, or diagonally?

- **a.** Base placement
- **b.** Base direction
- **c.** Base insertion
- **d.** Base reduction

____

43. A _____ is a type of wrap that uses one end paper folded in half over the hair ends like an envelope.

- **a.** basic permanent wrap
- **b.** curvature permanent wrap
- **c.** bricklay permanent wrap
- **d.** bookend wrap

____

44. A _____ is a wrapping pattern in which all the rods within a panel move in the same direction and are positioned on equal-sized bases.

- **a.** basic permanent wrap
- **b.** croquignole perm wrap
- **c.** double-rod wrap
- **d.** bookend wrap

____

45. Which of these are usually classified as a lye-based relaxer?

- **a.** Metal hydroxide relaxers
- **b.** Carbonate hydroxide relaxers
- **c.** Sodium hydroxide relaxers
- **d.** Iron hydroxide relaxers

____

46. Which rods are equal in diameter along their entire length or curling area?

- **a.** Straight rods
- **b.** Loop rods
- **c.** Concave rods
- **d.** Convex rods

____

47. Which of these terms refers to the thickness or thinness of a liquid?

- **a.** Duration
- **b.** Viscosity
- **c.** Intensity
- **d.** Amperage

____

48. The _____ is the tough exterior layer of the hair.
    a. cuticle   **c.** base
    b. medulla   **d.** cortex   ____

49. Which of these terms refers to the position of the rod in relation to its base section?
    a. Base altitude   **c.** Base direction
    b. Half off-base placement   **d.** Base placement   ____

50. A _____ is a type of wrap in which the hair is wrapped on one rod from the scalp to midway down the hair shaft, and another rod is used to wrap the remaining hair strand in the same direction.
    a. spiral perm wrap
    b. double flat wrap
    c. piggyback wrap
    d. bricklay permanent wrap   ____

51. Which of these stops the action of the waving solution and rebuilds the hair into its new curly form?
    a. Lanthionization   **c.** Hydroxidation
    b. Thio neutralization   **d.** Peptide concentration   ____

52. Long chains of amino acids joined together by peptide bonds are known as _____.
    a. neutralization chains   **c.** amino chains
    b. monopeptide chains   **d.** polypeptide chains   ____

53. The process by which hydroxide relaxers permanently straighten hair is called _____.
    a. lanthionization   **c.** normalization
    b. permanent waving   **d.** disulfide bonding   ____

54. Hydrogen bonds can be broken by _____.
    a. only water   **c.** either water or heat
    b. only heat   **d.** neither water nor heat   ____

55. The reducing agent used in permanent waving solutions is commonly referred to as _____.
    a. hydroxide   **c.** sulfate
    b. thio   **d.** disulfide   ____

56. Manufacturers add an alkalizing agent to waving solutions because the acid in the solutions _____.
    a. swells the hair
    b. penetrates into the cortex
    c. both swells the hair and penetrates into the cortex
    d. does not swell the hair or penetrate into the cortex ____

57. A pH of 7.0 is _____ than the pH of hair.
    a. 10 times more alkaline   c. 10 times more acidic
    b. 100 times more alkaline   d. 100 times more acidic ____

58. Most of the acid waves found in today's salons have a pH between _____.
    a. 7.8 and 8.2   c. 3.8 and 4.2
    b. 9.5 and 10.5   d. 4.5 and 5.5 ____

59. Which of the following is not considered a main component of an exothermic wave?
    a. Permanent waving solution   c. Activator
    b. Neutralizer   d. Concentrator ____

60. An endothermic chemical reaction is one that absorbs _____ from its surroundings.
    a. moisture   c. heat
    b. energy   d. light ____

61. Which type of perm is recommended for extremely porous hair?
    a. True acid wave   c. Ammonia-free wave
    b. Exothermic wave   d. Alkaline wave ____

62. What is the most common neutralizer?
    a. Ammonia   c. Sodium chloride
    b. Hydrogen peroxide   d. Distilled water ____

63. When rinsing the hair after the recommended processing time has elapsed, it is recommended that you _____.
    a. never rinse for longer than 20 seconds
    b. make sure the hair is still moderately moist before neutralizing
    c. smell the hair to determine if it still smells like perming solution
    d. aggressively blot the hair ____

64. Japanese thermal straightening _____.
  a. is a recommended service for extremely curly hair
  b. usually takes about 30 minutes
  c. is appropriate for all color-treated hair
  d. is sometimes called thermal reconditioning   ____

65. Mild-strength relaxers are formulated for _____.
  a. normal hair texture with a medium natural curl
  b. fine, color-treated, or damaged hair
  c. very coarse, extremely curly hair
  d. resistant hair with little damage   ____

CHAPTER 21 HAIRCOLORING

1. The layer of the hair that gives the hair the majority of its strength and elasticity is the _____.
   a. cortex
   b. cuticle
   c. follicle
   d. medulla ____

2. In individual hair strands, hair texture is determined by the _____.
   a. density
   b. porosity
   c. diameter
   d. length ____

3. If the cuticle is lifted, allowing the hair to take color quickly, the hair is said to have _____.
   a. average porosity
   b. no porosity
   c. low porosity
   d. high porosity ____

4. Haircolor levels are arranged on a scale from _____.
   a. 1 to 5
   b. 1 to 10
   c. 1 to 100
   d. 0 to 14 ____

5. Hair color tones can be described as _____.
   a. warm, neutral, or hot
   b. warm, cool, or neutral
   c. cool, neutral, or even
   d. cool, warm, or primary ____

6. Warm tones that are described as sandy or tan are considered _____.
   a. natural
   b. primary
   c. artificial
   d. cool ____

7. Which color will help balance orange tones in the hair?
   a. Violet
   b. Gold
   c. Green
   d. Blue ____

8. Pure or fundamental colors that cannot be created by combining other colors are called _____.
   a. level colors
   b. secondary colors
   c. primary colors
   d. cool colors ____

9. The strongest and only cool primary color
   is _____.
   a. green   c. red
   b. yellow   d. blue   ____

10. Red added to blue-based colors will cause them to
    appear _____.
    a. lighter   c. golden
    b. darker   d. yellow   ____

11. A _____ color is achieved by mixing a secondary
    color and its neighboring primary color.
    a. warm   c. complementary
    b. tertiary   d. base   ____

12. In traditional color theory, when all three primary colors
    are present in equal proportions, the resulting color
    is _____ depending on the saturation of the pigment.
    a. white or gray
    b. rust or brown
    c. black or dark muddy gray
    d. green or muddy blue   ____

13. A primary and secondary color positioned directly
    opposite each other on the color wheel are
    considered _____.
    a. base colors   c. opposing colors
    b. tertiary colors   d. complementary colors   ____

14. Temporary haircolor pigment molecules do not penetrate
    the cuticle layer because they have _____ pigment
    molecules.
    a. strong   c. small
    b. weak   d. large   ____

15. Traditional semipermanent haircolor only lasts _____,
    depending on how frequently the hair is shampooed.
    a. four to six days   c. eight to ten weeks
    b. four to six weeks   d. two to three weeks   ____

16. Which type of haircolor is formulated to deposit but not
    lighten color?
    a. Demipermanent haircolor
    b. Permanent haircolor
    c. Semipermanent haircolor
    d. Temporary haircolor   ____

122

17. Which type of haircolor lightens and deposits color at the same time and in a single process because it is more alkaline than demipermanent colors and is usually mixed with a higher-volume developer?
   a. Temporary haircolor
   b. Permanent haircolor
   c. Semipermanent haircolor
   d. Natural haircolor ____

18. To provide maximum lift in a one-step color service, which volume of peroxide is recommended?
   a. 20-volume peroxide
   b. 15-volume peroxide
   c. 30-volume peroxide
   d. 40-volume peroxide ____

19. During the decolorizing process, natural hair can go through as many as _____.
   a. two stages
   b. one stage
   c. ten stages
   d. five stages ____

20. Overlapping color can cause breakage and create _____.
   a. uniform color
   b. a line of demarcation
   c. a barrier line
   d. streaking ____

21. The three forms of hair lighteners are _____.
   a. oil, powder, and cream
   b. oil, cream, and lotion
   c. powder, foam, and oil
   d. cream, powder, and foam ____

22. In _____, selected strands are picked up from a narrow section of hair with a zigzag motion of the comb, and lightener or color is applied only to these strands.
   a. slicing
   b. baliage
   c. free-form technique
   d. weaving ____

23. For clients with 80 to 100 percent gray, which haircolor is generally more flattering?
   a. A blond shade
   b. A medium-brown shade
   c. A dark-brown shade
   d. A red shade ____

24. To cover unpigmented hair on a salt-and-pepper head, the color formulation should be _____ than the natural level.
   a. one level darker
   b. one to two levels lighter
   c. four levels lighter
   d. two levels darker ____

25. The process of treating gray or very resistant hair to allow for better penetration of color is known as _____.
    a. formulating   **c.** pre-softening
    b. unpigmenting   **d.** pre-lightening   ____

26. When performing a lightener retouch, new growth is lightened _____.
    a. first   **c.** last
    b. second   **d.** not at all   ____

27. To produce a haircolor that looks natural, how many primary colors must be present?
    a. One   **c.** Three
    b. Two   **d.** Four   ____

28. The best way to obtain pale blond results is to use _____.
    a. temporary haircolor
    b. pure bleach
    c. single process blonding
    d. double-process blonding   ____

29. When hair is violet, it is recommended that you use _____ to balance it.
    a. orange   **c.** yellow
    b. green   **d.** red   ____

30. When hair is blue, it is recommended that you use _____ to balance it.
    a. orange   **c.** red
    b. violet   **d.** green   ____

31. Selecting _____ base colors creates brighter colors.
    a. cooler   **c.** neutral
    b. warm   **d.** soft   ____

32. Demipermanent haircolor _____ color.
    a. both deposits and lifts
    b. neither deposits nor lifts
    c. lifts but does not deposit
    d. deposits but does not lift   ____

33. During a haircolor consultation, you should _____.
    a. look at the client in the mirror
    b. look at the client directly
    c. look only at the client's hair
    d. avoid looking at the client ____

34. Traditional semipermanent, demipermanent, and permanent haircolor products that are used primarily on pre-lightened hair to achieve pale and delicate colors are _____.
    a. lighteners   c. toners
    b. bleaches   d. tints ____

35. When performing a patch test, which color should you use?
    a. The same color that will be used for the haircolor service
    b. A shade slightly darker than the client's natural shade
    c. A shade slightly lighter than the client's natural shade
    d. The lightest shade available ____

36. Hair that has previously received a color service will have _____.
    a. no porosity
    b. a greater degree of porosity
    c. a typical level of porosity
    d. much less porosity ____

37. Underlightened hair will appear to have more _____ than the intended color.
    a. violet, green, or blue   c. red or green
    b. orange or blue   d. red, yellow, or orange ____

38. The term _____, or hue, refers to the balance of color.
    a. shade   c. intensity
    b. tone   d. level ____

39. Which of these is a coloring technique that requires two separate procedures in which the hair is pre-lightened before the depositing color is applied?
    a. Cap technique
    b. Reverse highlighting
    c. Baliage
    d. Double-process application ____

40. The melanin that gives blond and red colors to hair is called _____.
a. eumelanin
b. mixed melanin
c. pheomelanin
d. cyanomelanin

_____

41. The powdered persulfate salts added to the haircolor to increase its lightening ability are called _____.
a. activators
b. toners
c. highlighters
d. fillers

_____

42. The technique called _____ refers to a combination of equal parts of a prepared permanent color mixture and shampoo used during the last five minutes of a haircolor service and worked through the hair to refresh the ends.
a. decolorizing
b. highlighting
c. shampoo oxidation
d. a soap cap

_____

43. Which of these terms refers to varying degrees of warmth exposed during a permanent color or lightening process?
a. Overtone
b. Contributing pigment
c. Hue
d. Level

_____

44. Which of these is a technique of coloring strands of hair darker than the natural color?
a. Reverse highlighting
b. Two-step coloring
c. Bleaching
d. Highlighting

_____

45. What is the unit of measurement used to identify the lightness or darkness of a color?
a. Hue
b. Tone
c. Intensity
d. Level

_____

46. Predisposition test, also known as a _____, identifies a possible allergy in a client.
a. strand test
b. patch test
c. color level test
d. allergy test

_____

47. A(n) _____ is a chemical compound that lightens hair by dispersing, dissolving, and decolorizing the natural hair pigment.
a. toner
b. soap cap
c. lightener
d. activator

_____

48. Which of these measures the concentration and strength of hydrogen peroxide?

    a. Intensity   **c.** Level

    b. Volume   **d.** Tone   ____

49. Colors obtained from the leaves or bark of plants are called _____.

    a. earth tone haircolors   **c.** ecocolors

    b. biocolors   **d.** natural haircolors   ____

50. A _____ is a non-ammonia color that adds shine and tone to the hair.

    a. gradual haircolor   **c.** glaze

    b. pheomelanin   **d.** filler   ____

51. The term _____ means it is difficult for moisture or chemicals to penetrate the hair.

    a. baliage   **c.** resistant

    b. demipermanent   **d.** level   ____

52. Which of the following is used to recondition damaged, overly porous hair and equalize porosity so that the hair accepts the color evenly from strand to strand and from scalp to ends?

    a. Conditioner filler   **c.** Glaze

    b. Color filler   **d.** Activator   ____

53. Which of these is an oxidizing agent that, when mixed with an oxidation haircolor, supplies the necessary oxygen gas to develop the color molecules and create a change in natural hair color?

    a. Hydrogen peroxide developer   **c.** Toner

    b. Permanent haircolor   **d.** Gradual haircolor   ____

54. A _____ is used to equalize porosity and deposit color in one application to provide a uniform contributing pigment on pre-lightened hair.

    a. conditioner filler   **c.** color filler

    b. toning glaze   **d.** developer   ____

55. Which of these is a process that involves taking a narrow, $\frac{1}{8}$-inch (0.3 centimeter) section of hair by making a straight part at the scalp, positioning the hair over the foil, and applying lightening or color?

    a. Decolorizing   **c.** Highlighting

    b. Baliage   **d.** Slicing   ____

56. The system for understanding color relationships is called _____.
   a. the color wheel   **c.** chromatics
   b. the law of color   **d.** the rule of tones   ____

57. The term _____ refers to the first time the hair is colored.
   a. virgin application   **c.** pre-service
   b. proto-application   **d.** retouch   ____

58. Which type of melanin lends black and brown colors to hair?
   a. Mixed melanin   **c.** Pheomelanin
   b. Cyanomelanin   **d.** Eumelanin   ____

59. A quick lightener, also known as _____, is a powdered lightener.
   a. a pre-softener
   b. a reverse highlighter
   c. an off-the-scalp lightener
   d. a toner   ____

60. Haircolors containing metal salts that change hair color gradually by progressive buildup and exposure to air, creating a dull, metallic appearance, are called _____.
   a. sodium haircolors   **c.** tertiary haircolors
   b. progressive haircolors   **d.** aniline derivatives   ____

61. A(n) _____ is a test performed to determine how the hair will react to the color formula and how long the formula should be left on the hair.
   a. strand test   **c.** base test
   b. patch test   **d.** activation test   ____

62. When identifying natural levels for a haircolor service, your most valuable tool is the _____.
   a. finishing comb   **c.** vent brush
   b. LED lamp   **d.** color wheel   ____

63. The medium primary color is _____.
   a. red   **c.** yellow
   b. blue   **d.** violet   ____

64. Which type of color adds subtle color results?
- **a.** Demipermanent haircolor
- **c.** Permanent haircolor
- **b.** Semipermanent haircolor
- **d.** Temporary haircolor   ____

65. Which of these is a role of the alkalizing ingredient in permanent haircolor?
- **a.** To decrease the penetration of the dye within the hair
- **b.** To prevent the lightening action of peroxide
- **c.** To raise the cuticle of the hair
- **d.** To coat the hair without penetrating it   ____

66. Henna is an example of _____.
- **a.** metallic haircolor
- **c.** temporary haircolor
- **b.** natural haircolor
- **d.** highlighting haircolor   ____

67. What is the standard hydrogen peroxide volume?
- **a.** 10-volume
- **c.** 30-volume
- **b.** 20-volume
- **d.** 40-volume   ____

68. A release statement is not considered to be _____.
- **a.** protection for the school or salon in case of accidents
- **b.** useful in explaining to clients the risk involved in a chemical service
- **c.** required for most forms of malpractice insurance
- **d.** a legally binding contract   ____

69. Semipermanent colors _____.
- **a.** lighten color
- **c.** deposit color
- **b.** contain oxidizers
- **d.** remove color   ____

70. The technique that involves pulling clean, dry strands of hair through a perforated cap with a thin plastic or metal hook is called _____.
- **a.** weaving
- **c.** cap technique
- **b.** hooking technique
- **d.** slicing   ____

71. A _____ contains no ammonia, requires no developer, and is gentle on the scalp and hair.
- **a.** non-oxidative toner
- **c.** pre-softener
- **b.** lightener
- **d.** toner   ____

72. Colors prepared by combining permanent haircolor, hydrogen peroxide, and shampoo are called _____.
- **a.** mixed shampoos
- **c.** highlighting shampoos
- **b.** highlighting colors
- **d.** permanent shampoos   ____

73. Coating compounds such as hair sprays, styling agents, and some conditioners can interfere with _____.
a. hair conditioning
b. color penetration
c. hair porosity
d. hair elasticity

____

74. A daily shampoo and blowdry, an occasional permanent wave, or a few days in the pool can cause the artificial pigment in red hair to _____.
a. solidify and strengthen
b. become more vibrant
c. stabilize and activate
d. oxidize and fade

____

75. A _____ consistency provides the best control during the application of lightener as part of a double-process haircoloring service.
a. creamy
b. watery
c. powdery
d. very thick

____

22 HAIR REMOVAL

1. During the client consultation, all clients should complete a client intake form that discloses _____ medications.
   a. topical
   b. oral
   c. both oral and topical
   d. allergy medicines

   ____

2. An absolute requirement for laser hair removal is that the hair being removed must be _____.
   a. lighter than the surrounding skin
   b. darker than the surrounding skin
   c. in the anagen phase
   d. in the catagen phase

   ____

3. The tool used, particularly to remove unwanted hair at the nape of the neck is _____.
   a. tweezers
   b. an electric clipper
   c. shears
   d. a straight razor

   ____

4. The natural arch of the eyebrow follows the _____.
   a. orbital bone
   b. frontal bone
   c. mandible bone
   d. frontal muscle

   ____

5. The recommended time between waxings is generally _____.
   a. one week
   b. two to four weeks
   c. four to six weeks
   d. six to eight weeks

   ____

6. If redness or swelling occurs after a waxing treatment, calm and soothe the skin with the application of _____ and cool compresses.
   a. aloe gel
   b. a moisturizing lotion
   c. rubbing alcohol
   d. an astringent

   ____

7. Threading, also known as _____, is a temporary hair removal method whereby cotton thread is twisted and rolled along the surface of the skin, entwining the hair in the thread and lifting it from the follicle.
   a. stringing
   b. rolling
   c. stretching
   d. banding
   ____

8. An advantage of sugaring is that it can be used to remove hair as short as _____ long.
   a. $\frac{1}{8}$-inch
   b. $\frac{1}{4}$-inch
   c. $\frac{1}{2}$-inch
   d. $\frac{1}{3}$-inch
   ____

9. When heated wax is ready to be applied to the skin it should be warm but not hot and _____.
   a. be bubbling from the heat
   b. have a thick consistency, like peanut butter
   c. flow off the spatula as a liquid
   d. drip smoothly off the spatula
   ____

10. During a body waxing using soft wax, if wax strings and lands on the client in an area you do not wish to treat, you should remove it with _____.
    a. a cloth saturated with warm water
    b. a cloth saturated with rubbing alcohol
    c. a lotion designed to dissolve and remove wax
    d. astringent or toner
    ____

11. An epilator removes the hair from _____.
    a. the bottom of the follicle
    b. the middle of the follicle
    c. the top of the follicle
    d. all parts of the follicle
    ____

12. Which method of hair removal uses intense light to destroy the growth cells of the hair follicles?
    a. Tweezing
    b. Photoepilation
    c. Electrolysis
    d. Hirsutism
    ____

13. Which method of hair removal requires the removal of all the hair from the front and back of the bikini area?
    a. Sugaring
    b. Waxing
    c. Brazilian bikini waxing
    d. Threading
    ____

14. Which method of hair removal temporarily removes superfluous hair by dissolving it at the skin's surface?
    a. Threading
    b. Laser hair removal
    c. Electrolysis
    d. Depilatory
    ____

15. Which method of hair removal uses an electric current to destroy the growth cells of the hair?
    a. Photoepilation
    b. Electrolysis
    c. Laser hair removal
    d. Sugaring
    ____

16. Which of the following conditions is not considered a common contraindication for hair removal?
    a. Chronic migraines
    b. Recent cosmetic surgery
    c. Sunburn
    d. Pustules
    ____

17. Which of the following areas is less likely than the others to be an area requested by men for hair removal?
    a. The neck
    b. The feet
    c. The chest
    d. The back
    ____

18. When performing a patch test for a depilatory, how long should the product be left on the skin?
    a. Thirty to sixty seconds
    b. Two to three minutes
    c. Five to seven minutes
    d. Seven to ten minutes
    ____

19. Which of these is the appropriate hair removal procedure for a client's underarms?
    a. Cutting with scissors
    b. A depilatory
    c. Waxing
    d. Tweezing
    ____

20. Which part of the body is deemed inappropriate for tweezing?
    a. The tops of the feet
    b. The shoulders
    c. The bikini line
    d. The upper lip
    ____

21. If hair is more than _____ long, it should be trimmed before waxing.
    a. $\frac{1}{4}$-inch
    b. $\frac{1}{2}$-inch
    c. 1-inch
    d. $1\frac{1}{2}$-inches
    ____

22. Laser hair removal is most effective when used on follicles that are in the _____ phase.
    a. catagen
    b. telogen
    c. resting
    d. anagen
    ____

23. Another name for hirsuties is _____.
   a. hypertrichosis
   b. hypertrophy
   c. hyperhidrosis
   d. hypopigmentation   ____

24. Electrolysis involves the administration of an electric current with a very fine _____.
   a. set of round paddles
   b. short metal strip
   c. needle-shaped electrode
   d. rod-like electrode   ____

25. Photoepilation _____.
   a. has significant side effects
   b. requires the use of needles
   c. poses a significant risk of infection
   d. can clear 50 to 60 percent of hair in 12 weeks   ____

CHAPTER 23 FACIALS

1. When removing a cleanser from the eye area, it should be done with damp facial sponges or cotton pads _____.
   a. in upward and outward movements
   b. in down and across movements
   c. with back-and-forth movements
   d. in circular movements ____

2. When performing a skin analysis with a magnifying lamp, the first thing the technician should look for is the presence or absence of _____.
   a. closed comedones   c. evaporated cells
   b. visible pores   d. oily skin areas ____

3. Skin that may be flaky or dry looking, with small, fine lines and wrinkles is characterized as _____.
   a. dehydrated   c. normal
   b. oily   d. sensitive ____

4. Oily skin or skin that produces too much sebum may appear shiny or greasy and have _____.
   a. even pore distribution   c. flakes
   b. small pores   d. large pores ____

5. When a follicle becomes clogged, resulting in an infection of the follicle, it is caused by a type of acne bacteria called _____.
   a. hydrating bacteria   c. anaerobic bacteria
   b. sebumatic bacteria   d. aerobic bacteria ____

6. Red pimples that do not have a pus head are referred to as _____.
   a. elastin pimples   c. pustules
   b. acne papules   d. moles ____

7. Which of these is a skin condition caused by sun exposure or hormone imbalances resulting in dark blotches of color on areas of the skin?
   - **a.** Hypertrichosis
   - **b.** Acne
   - **c.** Dehydration
   - **d.** Hyperpigmentation
   _____

8. Which of these is a chronic hereditary disorder indicated by constant or frequent facial blushing?
   - **a.** Rosacea
   - **b.** Tinea
   - **c.** Acne
   - **d.** Albinism
   _____

9. Cosmetology professionals must not perform treatments that remove beyond the _____.
   - **a.** subcutaneous tissue
   - **b.** stratum dermis
   - **c.** stratum corneum
   - **d.** dermal layer
   _____

10. Which of these is a gentle, natural occurring exfoliation acid that helps dissolve the bonds and intercellular cement between cells?
    - **a.** Alpha hydroxy acid
    - **b.** Microdermabrasion
    - **c.** Enzyme peel
    - **d.** Cryogenic acid
    _____

11. A _____ is a concentrated product designed to penetrate the skin and treat various skin conditions and is applied under a moisturizer or sunscreen.
    - **a.** gommage
    - **b.** tonic
    - **c.** mask
    - **d.** serum
    _____

12. The thin, open-meshed fabric of loosely woven cotton that is used to hold the mask on the face is called

    _____.
    - **a.** mask padding
    - **b.** microsilk
    - **c.** gauze
    - **d.** a pledget
    _____

13. Which massage movement is a light, continuous stroking movement applied in a slow, rhythmic manner with the fingers or palms?
    - **a.** Tapotement
    - **b.** Pétrissage
    - **c.** Kneading
    - **d.** Effleurage
    _____

14. Which of these is a form of pétrissage in which the tissue is grasped, gently lifted, and spread out?
    - **a.** Fulling
    - **b.** Rolling
    - **c.** Friction
    - **d.** Chucking
    _____

15. What is the most stimulating form of massage that should be applied with care and discretion?
    a. Fulling   **c.** Tapotement
    b. Stroking   **d.** Chucking   ____

16. The point on the skin that covers the muscle where pressure or stimulation will cause contraction of the muscle is referred to as the _____.
    a. insertion point   **c.** origin point
    b. motor point   **d.** connection point   ____

17. When using a brushing machine to perform an exfoliation, the skin should be treated with a(n) _____.
    a. thin layer of cleanser or moisturizer
    b. fairly thick layer of cleanser or moisturizer
    c. strong toner
    d. astringent lotion   ____

18. The process of softening and emulsifying hardened sebum stuck in the follicles is called _____.
    a. massage therapy   **c.** desincrustation
    b. passive therapy   **d.** electrotherapy   ____

19. The process of using galvanic current to enable water-soluble products that contain ions to penetrate the skin is called _____.
    a. iontophoresis   **c.** cathodization
    b. micropenetration   **d.** extraction   ____

20. The therapeutic use of plant aromas for beauty and health treatment is _____.
    a. oil therapy   **c.** electrotherapy
    b. scentification   **d.** aromatherapy   ____

21. If you use harsh scrubs on sensitive skin, it can _____.
    a. aggravate redness
    b. affect the circulation
    c. cause severe blistering
    d. cause bruising   ____

22. Sun-damaged skin is often confused with _____.
    a. sensitive skin   **c.** aging skin
    b. inflamed skin   **d.** hypopigmented skin

23. Salon AHA exfoliants should never be used unless the client has been using 10 percent AHA products at home for _____ prior to the higher concentration salon treatment, has no contraindications for exfoliation treatment, and is using a daily facial sunscreen product.

    a. at least one week
    b. at least two weeks
    c. no more than one week
    d. no more than two weeks   ____

24. Compared to day-use products, night treatments are usually _____.

    a. lighter   **c.** less intensive
    b. equal in weight   **d.** more intensive   ____

25. One of the biggest benefits of massage is that it _____.

    a. causes clients' skin to tense, opening the pores
    b. eliminates the need for treatment products
    c. increases product absorption
    d. decreases the conditioning effect of treatment products   ____

26. Clay-based masks are oil-absorbing cleansing masks that have an exfoliating and _____ effect on oily and combination skin.

    a. smoothing   **c.** moisturizing
    b. astringent   **d.** loosening   ____

27. Alginate masks are often _____ based.

    a. seaweed   **c.** sand
    b. aloe   **d.** vegetable   ____

28. Ingredients that attract water are known as _____.

    a. humectants   **c.** serums
    b. emollients   **d.** astringents   ____

29. A(n) _____ is a hair follicle impacted with solidified sebum and dead cell buildup that appears as small bumps just underneath the skin's surface.

    a. ostium   **c.** open comedone
    b. gommage   **d.** closed comedone   ____

30. Which type of mask contains special crystals of gypsum?

    a. Paraffin wax mask   **c.** Cream mask
    b. Modelage mask   **d.** Friction mask   ____

31. Which of these terms refers to a lack of lipids?
    a. Exfoliant
    b. Couperose
    c. Alipidic
    d. Prolipidic
    ____

32. Lotions that help rebalance the pH and remove remnants of cleanser from the skin are called _____.
    a. serums
    b. toners
    c. moisturizers
    d. exfoliants
    ____

33. A(n) _____ is an applicator for directing the electric current from a machine to the client's skin.
    a. electrode
    b. amperage
    c. wringer
    d. ampoule
    ____

34. The opening of a follicle is called the _____.
    a. anode
    b. hackle
    c. ostium
    d. follicle end
    ____

35. Which of these is a type of chemical exfoliant that works by dissolving keratin protein in the surface cells of the skin?
    a. Microdermabrasion
    b. Tapotement
    c. Desincrustation
    d. Enzyme peel
    ____

36. A(n) _____ is an individual dose of serum contained in a small vial.
    a. ampoule
    b. cathode
    c. ostium
    d. anode
    ____

37. The rapid shaking of the body part while the balls of the fingertips are pressed firmly on the point of application is called _____.
    a. hacking
    b. vibration
    c. slapping
    d. pétrissage
    ____

38. Products used to physically remove dead cell buildup are called _____.
    a. steamers
    b. electrodes
    c. mechanical exfoliants
    d. chemical exfoliants
    ____

39. The manual or mechanical manipulation of the body by rubbing, gently pinching, kneading, tapping, and other movements is called _____.
    a. telangiectasias
    b. massage
    c. iontophoresis
    d. microcurrent
    ____

40. Which of these terms refers to a condition that requires avoiding certain treatments, procedures, or products to prevent undesirable side effects?
   a. Effleurage
   c. Compensation
   b. Counter-treatment
   d. Contraindication   ____

41. A(n) _____ is a peeling cream that is rubbed off of the skin.
   a. alpha hydroxy acid
   c. gommage
   b. cleansing milk
   d. humectant   ____

42. Which of these is a condition in which areas of the skin have distended capillaries and diffuse redness?
   a. Couperose
   c. Albinism
   b. Iontophoresis
   d. Hyperpigmentation   ____

43. Electrical treatments are contraindicated on clients _____.
   a. who take isotretinoin
   b. who take Differin®
   c. with asthma
   d. with metal bone pins in the body   ____

44. The cosmetologist should avoid wearing which type of jewelry while administering a facial treatment?
   a. Earrings
   c. A necklace
   b. Rings
   d. An anklet   ____

45. Mild exfoliation will _____.
   a. make the skin more oily
   b. decrease the skin's moisture content
   c. decrease elasticity
   d. reduce hyperpigmentation   ____

46. Moisturizers for oily skin are most often in _____ form.
   a. lotion
   c. powder
   b. gel
   d. spray   ____

47. Modelage masks _____ and are very beneficial for dry, mature skin.
   a. are recommended for oily skin
   b. increase blood circulation
   c. should be applied to the lower neck
   d. are appropriate for clients with hypertension   ____

48. When performing pétrissage _____.
   a. your movements should be confined to the face and neck
   b. you should apply a great deal of pressure
   c. you lift, squeeze, and press the tissue
   d. your movements should be jerky   ____

49. Which type of massage involves grasping the flesh firmly in one hand and moving the hand up and down along the bone while the other hand keeps the arm or leg in a steady position?
   a. Wringing   c. Rolling
   b. Chucking   d. Tapotement   ____

50. Hacking is performed with which part of the hands?
   a. The fingertips   c. The palms
   b. The backs   d. The edges   ____

24 FACIAL MAKEUP

1. A _____ foundation provides heavier coverage and is usually intended for drier, more mature skin types.
   - **a.** water-based
   - **b.** cream
   - **c.** powder
   - **d.** gel
   _____

2. A _____ works well to apply and blend foundation, cream or powder blush, pressed powder, or concealer.
   - **a.** spatula
   - **b.** sponge
   - **c.** cotton pad
   - **d.** cotton swab
   _____

3. A _____ is produced when a product that is lighter than the client's skin tone is placed on the high planes of the face.
   - **a.** base
   - **b.** contour
   - **c.** matte finish
   - **d.** highlight
   _____

4. To clean professional makeup brushes, the brush should always be held under running water with the ferrule _____.
   - **a.** pointing outward
   - **b.** pointing upward
   - **c.** pointing downward
   - **d.** removed
   _____

5. To accurately interpret a client's beauty concerns, each makeup session must start with _____.
   - **a.** a consultation
   - **b.** an analysis
   - **c.** an evaluation
   - **d.** an appraisal
   _____

6. Which eye color is considered neutral and enhances any makeup color?
   - **a.** Green
   - **b.** Blue
   - **c.** Brown
   - **d.** Hazel
   _____

7. In eye makeup, a contour color is applied to _____ unwanted fullness/puffiness, contour the crease, or define the lash line.
   - **a.** maximize
   - **b.** soften
   - **c.** accentuate
   - **d.** minimize
   _____

8. What face shape has a greater length in proportion to its width than the square or round face?
   a. Triangular
   c. Oblong
   b. Diamond
   d. Round
   ____

9. To minimize a small, flat nose, a lighter foundation is applied _____.
   a. on the cheeks and sides of the nose, ending at the tip
   b. down the center of the nose, ending at the tip
   c. on the sides of the nose and nostrils
   d. onto the sides of the nose and into the laugh lines
   ____

10. The ideal eyebrow shape is positioned along three lines, with the second line running from the outer circle of the iris _____.
    a. upward
    c. outward
    b. inward
    d. downward
    ____

11. When red is _____ -based, it is cool.
    a. orange
    c. gold
    b. yellow
    d. blue
    ____

12. Creating _____ minimizes prominent facial features.
    a. highlights
    c. bright colors
    b. a shadow
    d. contours
    ____

13. What is the primary goal of makeup application?
    a. To cover up any wrinkles or blemishes
    b. To remake the client's image according to an ideal standard
    c. To add a great deal of color to the client's face
    d. To emphasize the client's most attractive features
    ____

14. If the client has close-set eyes, it is recommended that you apply a thin layer of light concealer _____.
    a. up from the top of the eyes
    b. to the outer corners of the eyes
    c. to the inner corners of the eyes
    d. down from the lower edge of the eyes
    ____

15. If the client has a square face, it is recommended that you _____.
    a. create a high arch on the ends of the eyebrows
    b. make the eyebrows almost straight
    c. widen the distance between the eyebrows
    d. trim the outer edges of the eyebrows
    ____

16. Which type of cosmetic is used to define the eyes?
  a. Mascara
  c. Eyeliner
  b. Brow pencil
  d. Eye shadow
  _____

17. Which of the following is used to hide dark eye circles, hyperpigmentation, distended capillaries, and other imperfections?
  a. Face powder
  c. Cake makeup
  b. Concealer
  d. Greasepaint
  _____

18. Heavy makeup primarily used for theatrical purposes is known as _____.
  a. cake makeup
  c. concealer
  b. foundation
  d. greasepaint
  _____

19. Which of the following is also known as base makeup?
  a. Foundation
  c. Cheek color
  b. Color primer
  d. Lip liner
  _____

20. The most common use of _____ outside the theater is to cover scars and uneven pigmentation.
  a. color primer
  c. mascara
  b. cake makeup
  d. face powder
  _____

21. Which of the following is used primarily to add color to the cheeks?
  a. Greasepaint
  c. Foundation
  b. Color primer
  d. Blush
  _____

22. Which of the following is a cosmetic preparation used to darken, define, and thicken the eyelashes?
  a. Eye shadow
  c. Mascara
  b. Eyeliner
  d. Concealer
  _____

23. Which of the following is applied to the skin before foundation to disguise less than perfect skin and actually neutralize skin discolorations?
  a. Primer
  c. Cheek color
  b. Cake makeup
  d. Face powder
  _____

24. Which of the following is a cosmetic used to accentuate the eye shape and compliment eye color?
  a. Mascara
  c. Eyeliner
  b. Eye shadow
  d. Brow powder
  _____

25. Lip color is available in many forms, which are a mixture of oils, waxes, and pigments known as _____ or color dyes.

  a. tones   **c.** blots

  b. lakes   **d.** mattes   ____

26. Cosmetic products that do not contain ingredients that would clog the follicles, aggravating acne-prone skin, are called _____.

  a. acneic   **c.** noncomedogenic

  b. pustulic   **d.** comedogenic   ____

27. Loose powder is applied with a large powder brush or a _____.

  a. linen facecloth   **c.** cotton swab

  b. wooden pusher   **d.** disposable powder puff   ____

28. Oil-based eye makeup removers are generally used to remove _____ makeup and break down the latex glue used to apply false eyelashes.

  a. heavy, dramatic   **c.** light, classic

  b. light, natural   **d.** corrective   ____

29. Which type of brush has fine, tapered, firm bristles and is used to apply liquid liner or shadow to the lash line?

  a. Angle brush   **c.** Eyeliner brush

  b. Concealer brush   **d.** Brow brush   ____

30. Which type of lashes are separate artificial eyelashes that are applied to the base of the eyelashes one at a time?

  a. Strip lashes   **c.** Band lashes

  b. Individual lashes   **d.** Strand lashes   ____

31. While spray-on cleaners can be used to quickly clean brushes, they contain a high level of _____ and are not recommended for daily use.

  a. alcohol   **c.** acetone

  b. glycerin   **d.** mineral oil   ____

32. Matching shadow color with eye color creates a _____ with a less dramatic depth of contrast.

  a. flat matte   **c.** colorful palette

  b. dull appearance   **d.** monochromatic field   ____

33. Expression lines and wrinkles can be minimized with a _____ and foundation.
    a. highlighter
    b. glossy powder
    c. skin primer
    d. frosted cream   ____

34. What is the makeup goal for a heart-shaped face?
    a. To offset the shape of softening the hard angles
    b. To minimize the width of the forehead and increase the width of the jawline
    c. To create width at the forehead and slenderize the jawline
    d. To minimize the width of the outer cheekbone   ____

35. Skin that has a yellowish hue is known as _____ skin.
    a. ruddy
    b. flushed
    c. sallow
    d. translucent   ____

25 MANICURING

1. An adjustable lamp is attached to the manicuring table and should use a _____ incandescent bulb or a fluorescent bulb.
   a. 10- to 30-watt
   c. 70- to 90-watt
   b. 40- to 60-watt
   d. 100- to 120-watt ____

2. Fine-grit abrasives are designed for removing very fine scratches and _____.
   a. buffing and polishing
   c. aggressive buffing
   b. smoothing and refining
   d. shortening and shaping ____

3. Protein hardener is a combination of what two ingredients?
   a. Collagen and elastin
   b. Clear polish and protein
   c. Clear polish and formaldehyde
   d. Colored polish and elastin ____

4. Nail products should be removed from their respective containers using a _____ to prevent contamination of the products and the spread of disease.
   a. wooden pusher
   b. finger
   c. single-use plastic or metal spatula
   d. cotton swab ____

5. Which of the following products is designed to loosen and dissolve dead tissue on the nail plate?
   a. Moisturizing lotion
   c. Acetone remover
   b. Non-acetone remover
   d. Cuticle remover ____

6. The most successful nail polish application is achieved by using four coats including _____.
   a. two coats of polish color and two top coats
   b. two base coats, one coat of polish color, and one top coat
   c. one base coat, two coats of polish color, and one top coat
   d. one base coat, one coat of polish color, and two top coats ____

7. A standard manicuring table _____.
 a. is usually 16 to 21 inches wide
 b. is usually 24 to 36 inches long
 c. has no drawers or shelves
 d. does not require cleaning and disinfection _____

8. If a single client is going to receive both a manicure and a pedicure, how many sets of gloves will the cosmetologist need?
 a. None   **c.** Two
 b. One   **d.** Three _____

9. Disinfection containers come in many shapes, sizes, and materials and must have _____.
 a. a drain   **c.** a timer
 b. a tray   **d.** a lid _____

10. Which of the following products or supplies are kept in a place other than the supply tray?
 a. Polishes   **c.** Creams
 b. Electric nail polish dryer   **d.** Polish removers _____

11. Tiny, often unseen openings in the skin, which can allow microbes to enter the skin, leading to infection, are known as _____.
 a. microscopic injury   **c.** mini-damage
 b. macrotrauma   **d.** microtrauma _____

12. The best terry cloth towels for use in a personal service are _____.
 a. white   **c.** yellow
 b. gray   **d.** black _____

13. Soap is known to remove _____ of pathogenic microbes from the hands when hand washing is performed properly.
 a. nearly 50 percent   **c.** over 80 percent
 b. about 75 percent   **d.** over 90 percent _____

14. Compared to non-acetone removers, acetone-based removers _____.
 a. work faster but are poorer solvents
 b. work slower but are poorer solvents
 c. work faster removing polish and evaporate rapidly
 d. work slower but are better solvents _____

15. Which of the following is designed to seal the surface of the skin around the nail?
    a. Nail oil
    b. Nail cream
    c. Nail lotion
    d. Acetone
    ____

16. Which of the following does not describe a colored coating applied to the natural nail plate?
    a. Nail lacquer
    b. Nail varnish
    c. Nail bleach
    d. Nail enamel
    ____

17. Nail hardeners can be applied _____.
    a. only before the base coat
    b. only as a top coat
    c. either before the base coat or as a top coat
    d. after an oil manicure
    ____

18. The purpose of massage in manicuring is the inducement of _____.
    a. stimulation
    b. metabolism
    c. circulation
    d. relaxation
    ____

19. A petroleum by-product that has excellent sealing properties to hold moisture in the skin is _____.
    a. lanolin
    b. paraffin
    c. glycerin
    d. sealant
    ____

20. A spa manicure requires extensive knowledge of _____.
    a. polish application
    b. pampering
    c. nail and skin care
    d. chemical-free products
    ____

21. Which of these terms refers to the tools used to perform your services?
    a. Implements
    b. Instruments
    c. Equipment
    d. Products
    ____

22. Which of these terms refers to age spots caused by ultraviolet light (UVA) from the sun?
    a. Hypotension
    b. Hypertension
    c. Hypopigmentation
    d. Hyperpigmentation
    ____

23. Which massage movement involves a succession of strokes in which the hands glide over an area of the body with varying degrees of pressure or contact?
    a. Pétrissage
    b. Effleurage
    c. Tapotement
    d. Vibration
    ____

24. Rubbing a file across the edge of another clean, unused file to remove the sharp edge is referred to as _____.
    a. file prepping
    b. sharpening
    c. filing
    d. buffing
    ____

25. Which implement is used to carefully trim away dead skin around the nails?
    a. Metal pusher
    b. Tweezers
    c. Nail nippers
    d. Nail clippers
    ____

26. Which massage movement involves rapid tapping or striking motions of the hands against the skin?
    a. Friction
    b. Pétrissage
    c. Effleurage
    d. Tapotement
    ____

27. Which implement is used to shorten the free edge quickly and efficiently?
    a. Nail nippers
    b. Nail clippers
    c. Nail file
    d. Buffer
    ____

28. Which method of massage incorporates various strokes that manipulate or press one layer of tissue over another?
    a. Vibration
    b. Tapotement
    c. Effleurage
    d. Friction
    ____

29. A service cushion must be _____ throughout the service.
    a. fully covered by a fresh, clean towel
    b. covered with plastic
    c. higher on the ends than in the middle
    d. placed behind the client's back
    ____

30. The wooden pusher is used to remove cuticle tissue from the nail plate, to clean under the free edge of the nail, or to _____.
    a. shorten the free edge
    b. remove implements from disinfectant solutions
    c. clean nails during hand washing
    d. apply products
    ____

31. Products that contain ingredients to reduce brittleness of the nail are _____.
    a. paraffin waxes
    b. nail strengtheners
    c. nail conditioners
    d. ridge fillers
    ____

32. The _____ nail has a square free edge that is rounded off at the corner edges.
   a. pointed
   c. square
   b. squoval
   d. oval
   _____

33. The nail shape that should be slightly tapered and usually should extend just a bit past the fingertip is the _____.
   a. pointed nail shape
   c. square nail shape
   b. round nail shape
   d. squoval nail shape
   _____

34. The _____ nail is a conservative shape that is thought to be attractive on most women's hands.
   a. oval
   c. squoval
   b. pointed
   d. square
   _____

35. Essential oils are extracted using various forms of _____ from seeds, bark, roots, leaves, wood, and/or resin of plants.
   a. withdrawal
   c. distillation
   b. extraction
   d. evaporation
   _____

CHAPTER 26 PEDICURING

1. When performing a foot massage during a pedicure, you should grasp the foot between your thumb and fingers at the _____.
   a. bottom of the foot
   b. heel area
   c. mid-tarsal area
   d. ankle area

   ____

2. Hot stones used in pedicures are smooth and typically _____.
   a. granite
   b. basalt
   c. quartz
   d. slate

   ____

3. Products designed to soften and smooth thickened tissue are _____.
   a. foot creams
   b. skin solvents
   c. callus softeners
   d. callus removers

   ____

4. Which massage technique is used most with a pedicure?
   a. Effleurage
   b. Pétrissage
   c. Tapotement
   d. Reflexology

   ____

5. Which of the following should never be placed in the foot bath with the client's feet?
   a. Solution
   b. Antiseptic
   c. Magnesium salt
   d. Disinfectant

   ____

6. The chair a cosmetologist uses when performing a pedicure _____.
   a. is usually high off the ground
   b. should be ergonomic
   c. must be inexpensive
   d. should be contemporary

   ____

7. A concentrated treatment product often composed of mineral clays, moisturizing agents, skin softeners, aromatherapy oils, botanical extracts, and/or other beneficial ingredients is _____.
   a. a mask
   b. an exfoliant
   c. an emollient
   d. a scrub

   ____

8. Exfoliating scrubs are usually _____ lotions that contain _____ as the exfoliating agent.
   a. oil-based / an abrasive
   c. emollient / crystals
   b. water-based / an abrasive
   d. glycerin / granules   _____

9. In order to be on time for the next client, you should be polishing _____ after beginning a one-hour pedicure.
   a. 10 to 15 minutes
   c. 45 to 50 minutes
   b. 30 to 35 minutes
   d. 50 to 55 minutes   _____

10. Reflexology practitioners believe that stimulating or pressing certain reflexes or points on the feet can _____ to the specified areas.
    a. reflect positive energy
    b. decrease blood flow
    c. cause significant discomfort
    d. reverse the signs of aging   _____

11. A paraffin bath _____.
    a. promotes circulation
    b. reduces product absorption
    c. increases inflammation
    d. cools the skin   _____

12. An organic acid that derives originally from the bark of willow trees is _____.
    a. potassium hydroxide
    c. salicylic acid
    b. urea
    d. distilled acid   _____

13. If a client books a standard pedicure and you discover that the feet are in unusually bad condition and will require more time than was scheduled, it is recommended that you _____.
    a. take as much time as necessary, even if it means that other clients must wait
    b. send the client home and tell her to book a longer appointment next time
    c. cancel the next few appointments to make time for the client
    d. tell the client you will do the best you can in the time schedule, but another pedicure may be needed   _____

14. Scaly feet commonly require _____ treatment in the salon.
    a. daily
    b. weekly
    c. monthly
    d. yearly
    ____

15. Massage given during manicures and pedicures definitely focuses on _____.
    a. draining lymphatic fluid
    b. muscle stimulation
    c. pain relief
    d. relaxation
    ____

16. Which of these implements is commonly known as a pedicure paddle?
    a. Foot file
    b. Nail rasp
    c. Curette
    d. Nail file
    ____

17. Which of these is a metal implement with a grooved edge used for filing and smoothing the edges of the nail plate?
    a. Nail clipper
    b. Nail nippers
    c. Nail rasp
    d. Curette
    ____

18. A _____ is a small scoop-shaped implement used for more efficient removal of debris from the nail folds, eponychium, and hyponychium areas.
    a. nail rasp
    b. curette
    c. nail brush
    d. tweezers
    ____

19. Many elderly clients have health issues that, when receiving pedicure services, require _____.
    a. extra time
    b. medical supervision
    c. exceptionally gentle care
    d. special products
    ____

20. Which implement must be used carefully to prevent trapping the skin of the toe in the jaws?
    a. Toenail nippers
    b. Rasp
    c. Finishing scissors
    d. Curette
    ____

21. How long are masks typically left on the client's skin?
    a. Five to ten minutes
    b. Ten to fifteen minutes
    c. Fifteen to twenty minutes
    d. Twenty to thirty minutes
    ____

22. If a client wants to drift off during a pedicure, it is recommended that you _____.
   a. try to engage the client in pleasant conversation
   b. start telling the client about the home care products that you offer
   c. allow the client the peace and tranquility they are seeking
   d. squeeze the client's foot gently to keep them awake ____

23. Clients should be warned not to shave their legs within _____ a pedicure.
   a. 24 hours after   **c.** 24 hours before
   b. 48 hours after   **d.** 48 hours before ____

24. Some improvements in the feet require more than one appointment in services referred to as a _____.
   a. set   **c.** series
   b. system   **d.** selection ____

25. Who bears the responsibility for ensuring that proper disinfection of the pedicure bath occurs?
   a. The technician
   b. The salon
   c. The client
   d. The salon and the technician ____

27 NAIL TIPS & WRAPS

1. A _____ is a plastic, pre-molded nail shaped from a tough polymer made from acrylonitrile butadiene styrene (ABS) plastic.
   a. nail wrap
   b. nail tip
   c. nail overlay
   d. nail adhesive _____

2. The shallow depression area of a nail tip is the _____ that serves as the point of contact with the nail plate.
   a. well
   b. contact
   c. applicator
   d. gelled _____

3. When securing the tip to the natural nail plate, it is recommended that you use the _____ technique.
   a. stop, hold, and release
   b. stop, rock, and hold
   c. rock, hold, and free
   d. rock, slide, and release _____

4. When blending a nail tip at the contact area, the fine- to medium-grit file or buffing block file should be kept _____.
   a. at a 45-degree angle against the nail plate
   b. at a 80-degree angle against the nail plate
   c. at a 15-degree angle against the nail plate
   d. flat to the nail as you blend the tip _____

5. The strongest wrap fabric is considered to be _____.
   a. silk
   b. paper
   c. fiberglass
   d. linen _____

6. The product that acts as the dryer that speeds up the hardening process of the wrap resin or adhesive overlay is _____.
   a. a heat spike
   b. an extender
   c. an activator
   d. a dehydrator _____

7. A substance used to remove surface moisture and tiny amounts of oil left on the natural nail plate is a _____.
   a. nail blender
   b. nail activator
   c. nail adhesive
   d. nail dehydrator _____

8. A piece of fabric cut to completely cover a crack or break in the nail is a _____.
   a. stress strip
   b. repair patch
   c. rebalance batch
   d. refill strip

   _____

9. To avoid damaging nail wraps when removing existing polish, use a(n) _____.
   a. acetone remover
   b. oil accelerator
   c. resin softener
   d. non-acetone remover

   _____

10. An implement similar to a nail clipper, designed for use on nail tips, is a _____.
    a. tip nipper
    b. tip cutter
    c. stress cutter
    d. tip buffer

    _____

11. Fabric wraps are the most popular type of nail wrap because of their _____.
    a. durability
    b. color
    c. price
    d. glossy shine

    _____

12. Gel adhesives are sometimes referred to as _____.
    a. activator
    b. overlays
    c. resin
    d. dehydrators

    _____

13. Which wraps are made from a very thin synthetic mesh with a loose weave?
    a. Fiberglass wraps
    b. Silk wraps
    c. Linen wraps
    d. Paper wraps

    _____

14. Which wraps are made from a thin natural material with a tight weave that becomes transparent when wrap resin is applied?
    a. Linen wraps
    b. Fiberglass wraps
    c. Paper wraps
    d. Silk wraps

    _____

15. Which wraps are quite simple to use, but do not have the strength and durability of fabric wraps?
    a. Linen wraps
    b. Silk wraps
    c. Paper wraps
    d. Fiberglass wraps

    _____

16. Which type of wraps are made from a closely woven, heavy material?
    a. Silk wraps
    b. Linen wraps
    c. Fiberglass wraps
    d. Paper wraps

    _____

17. Nail adhesives usually come in either a tube with a pointed applicator tip, a one-drop applicator, or as _____.

  a. a tub.
  c. a spray-on.
  b. a vial.
  d. a brush-on. ____

18. *Maintenance* is the term used for when a nail enhancement needs to be serviced after _____ or more weeks from the initial application of the nail enhancement product.

  a. one
  c. four
  b. two
  d. six ____

19. The structural correction of the nail during a nail wrap maintenance service to ensure its strength, shape, and durability is known as _____.

  a. a fill
  c. a rebalance
  b. a backfill
  d. an activation ____

20. To remove fabric wraps, you first soak them in acetone and then _____.

  a. gently and carefully slide them off with a wooden pusher
  b. gently scrub them off with steel wool
  c. carefully cut them off with nippers
  d. precisely cut them off with scissors ____

21. A layer of any kind of nail enhancement product that is applied over the natural nail and tip application for added strength is known as _____.

  a. an over-application
  c. a top strengthener
  b. a double wrap
  d. an overlay ____

22. The point where the free edge of the natural nail meets the tip and where the tip is adhered to the nail is called the _____.

  a. tip point
  c. position stop
  b. well connection
  d. free edge groove ____

23. A strip of fabric cut to $\frac{1}{8}$-inch (3.12 mm) in length and applied to strengthen a weak point in the nail is called a _____.

  a. repair patch
  c. strengthener strip
  b. stress strip
  d. rebalance ____

24. What method of wrap removal may lead to damage of the nail plate by pulling off layers of the natural nail and can break the seal of the remainder of the enhancement?
   a. Nipping it off
   b. Sliding it off
   c. Soaking it off
   d. Soaking and sliding it off   ____

25. Nail tips that are _____ require much less filing on the natural nail after application.
   a. well-less   **c.** free-form
   b. pre-cut   **d.** pre-beveled   ____

28 MONOMER LIQUID & POLYMER POWDER NAIL ENHANCEMENTS

1. Sculptured nails are created by combining a chemical known as monomer liquid mixed with _____ to form a nail enhancement.
   a. monomer powder
   b. polymer powder
   c. liquid powder
   d. molecular powder ____

2. As monomer liquid absorbs a polymer powder, the product formed at the tip of the brush is referred to as a _____.
   a. cup
   b. bead
   c. dot
   d. pledget ____

3. The initiator that is added to polymer powder is called _____.
   a. benzoyl peroxide
   b. catalyst peroxide
   c. sodium hydroxide
   d. hydrogen peroxide ____

4. To prevent product contamination, a dappen dish should have _____.
   a. a loosely fitting lid
   b. a large opening
   c. a tightly fitting lid
   d. an evaporation lid ____

5. For many salon-related applications, gloves made of _____ work best.
   a. nylon polymer powder
   b. hard plastic
   c. latex polymer
   d. nitrile polymer powder ____

6. The bead of product for shaping the free edge should have a _____.
   a. wet consistency
   b. dry consistency
   c. medium-to-dry consistency
   d. medium-to-wet consistency ____

7. Which types of nail primers are most often used today?
   a. Acid-based and acid-free primers
   b. Acid-based and nonacid primers
   c. Acid-based and dual acid primers
   d. Acid-free and nonacid primers ____

8. When applying nonacid and acid-free nail primer, the brush should hold enough product to treat how many nails?
   a. One or two
   b. Two or three
   c. Six
   d. Eight
   ____

9. After a service, what should you do with tiny amounts of used monomer liquid left in the dappen dish?
   a. Pour the monomer liquid back into the container.
   b. Pour the monomer liquid directly into a plastic bag.
   c. Wipe the dappen dish with a paper towel and place the monomer liquid in a plastic bag.
   d. Pour the monomer liquid directly down the drain.
   ____

10. The _____ is the area of the nail with the most strength.
    a. apex
    b. stress area
    c. sidewall
    d. eponychium
    ____

11. A properly-worn dust mask will protect you from _____.
    a. dust only
    b. vapors only
    c. dust and vapors
    d. odors and vapors
    ____

12. In the maintenance service, _____.
    a. the nail is made thicker
    b. the entire nail enhancement is made thicker
    c. the apex of the nail is filed away
    d. the entire nail enhancement is removed
    ____

13. Which of these statements about catalysts is correct?
    a. Catalysts slow down chemical reactions between monomer liquid and polymer powder.
    b. Catalysts are added to monomer liquid to control the set or curing time.
    c. Catalysts destroy the initiators.
    d. Catalysts work by preventing the initiators from activating.
    ____

14. Polymer powder is available in _____.
    a. clear form only
    b. white only
    c. white and pink
    d. many colors
    ____

15. Which of these refers to one unit called a molecule?
    a. Polymer
    b. Monomer
    c. Initiator
    d. Catalyst
    ____

16. Which of these is a substance formed by combining many small molecules into very long, chain-like structures?
    a. Apex
    b. Bead
    c. Monomer
    d. Polymer
    ____

17. A substance that will spring into action and cause monomer molecules to permanently link together into long polymer chains is _____.
    a. an initiator
    b. a catalyst
    c. a reactor
    d. a concentrator
    ____

18. A _____ is a bead created using equal amounts of liquid and powder.
    a. wet bead
    b. dry bead
    c. damp bead
    d. medium bead
    ____

19. A _____ is a bead created using twice as much liquid as powder.
    a. damp bead
    b. medium bead
    c. dry bead
    d. wet bead
    ____

20. A _____ is a bead created using one-and-a-half times more liquid than powder.
    a. medium bead
    b. damp bead
    c. wet bead
    d. dry bead
    ____

21. Which of these is placed under the free edge of the natural nail and is used as a guide to extend the nail enhancement beyond the fingertip for additional length?
    a. Sidewall
    b. Monomer brush
    c. Nail form
    d. Curing strut
    ____

22. The area where the natural nail grows beyond the finger and becomes the free edge is called the _____.
    a. stress area
    b. nail form
    c. apex
    d. lunula
    ____

23. The area that runs straight from the cuticle down the side or wall of the nail to the end of the extension is called the _____.
    a. lunula
    b. sidewall
    c. free edge
    d. apex
    ____

24. Methyl methacrylate (MMA) is not recommended for use on nails because they do not adhere well to the nail plate, the rigidity of the product can lead to serious natural nail damage, it is extremely difficult to remove, and _____.
    a. they are hard to break
    b. they make the natural nail stronger
    c. they require special products to dissolve
    d. the FDA says not to use it   ____

25. A process that joins together monomers to create very long polymer chains is known as _____.
    a. monomerization
    b. resolution
    c. polymerization reaction
    d. chain maintenance   ____

26. Which of these abrasives would be appropriate for finish filing, refining, and buffing?
    a. 100-grit   c. 240-grit
    b. 4,000-grit   d. 180-grit   ____

27. After a monomer liquid and polymer powder service, you should wipe the dappen dish clean with _____ before storing it in a dust-free location.
    a. acetone   c. hot water
    b. hydrogen peroxide   d. cold water   ____

28. Nail extension undersides should _____.
    a. always jut straight out
    b. always dip
    c. be even, matched on each nail
    d. have a rough texture   ____

29. The apex is usually _____.
    a. oval shaped and located on the thumb-side of the nail
    b. oval shaped and located in the center of the nail
    c. rectangular and located at the base of the nail
    d. round and located beneath the nail   ____

30. In general, odorless products must be used with a _____ mix ratio.
    a. dry   c. damp
    b. wet   d. medium   ____

31. The number of grains of sand on an abrasive file per square inch is known as _____.
  a. sand paper
  b. density
  c. texture
  d. grit ____

32. Any nail art that protrudes from the nail is known as _____.
  a. protrusion art
  b. surface art
  c. 3-D art
  d. built-in art ____

33. Designs inside a nail enhancement that are created when nail art is sandwiched between two layers of product while the nail enhancement is being formed are called _____.
  a. sandwich art
  b. inlaid designs
  c. layered designs
  d. a design sandwich ____

1. A(n) _____ is a short chain of monomer liquids that is often thick, sticky, and gel-like and is not long enough to be considered a polymer.
   a. post-polymer   **c.** oligomer
   b. methacrylate   **d.** resin   ____

2. What is the most common UV bulb on the market?
   a. Four-watt   **c.** Seven-watt
   b. Nine-watt   **d.** Twelve-watt   ____

3. Light cured gels are usually packaged in opaque pots or _____.
   a. glass jars   **c.** plastic bags
   b. clear plastic bottles **d.** squeeze tubes ____

4. The tacky surface left on the nail after a UV or LED gel has cured is called the _____ layer.
   a. inhibition   **c.** adhesion
   b. contour   **d.** primary   ____

5. A _____ is recommended to refine the surface contour for UV or LED gel nails.
   a. nonabrasive
   b. metal file
   c. medium or fine abrasive
   d. harsh or coarse abrasive   ____

6. Viscosity is the measurement of the _____ of a liquid and how the fluid flows.
   a. weight   **c.** volume
   b. thickness   **d.** opacity   ____

7. Which of these products is used to increase adhesion of UV or LED gels to the natural nail plate?
   a. Nail primer   **c.** Bonding gel
   b. Nail adhesive   **d.** Nail cleanser   ____

8. Introducing air into the gel as you apply it to the fingernail will _____.
   a. help prevent cracking
   b. help the gel to cure more evenly
   c. give the nail a shinier appearance
   d. reduce the strength of the cured gel   ____

9. Which of these is a thick-viscosity resin that allows the cosmetologist to build an arch and curve into the fingernail?
   a. Building gel   c. Pigmented gel
   b. Soft UV or LED gel   d. Bonding gel   ____

10. A chemical called _____ initiates the polymerization reaction.
    a. a chemoinitiator   c. a capacitor
    b. an oligomer   d. a photoinitiator   ____

11. When gel polish is finished curing, a _____ can be applied over it to create a high, lustrous shine.
    a. gel polish   c. bonding gel
    b. gloss gel   d. building gel   ____

12. Which of these UV or LED gels cannot be removed with a solvent?
    a. Hard UV and LED gels
    b. Soft UV and LED gel
    c. UV and LED self-leveling gels
    d. UV and LED gloss gel   ____

13. Which type of gel is also known as soakable gel?
    a. Building gel   c. Pigmented gel
    b. UV and LED gel polish   d. Soft UV and LED gel   ____

14. Light cured gels _____.
    a. have a strong odor
    b. do not file easily
    c. can be easy to maintain
    d. are difficult to apply   ____

15. A very thin-viscosity gel that is used as an alternative to traditional nail lacquers is _____.
    a. a pigmented gel   c. a gel polish
    b. a self-leveling gel   d. a lacquer gel   ____

16. There are many names for glossing gels, but they do not include which of the following?
    a. Sealing gel
    b. Layer gel
    c. Finishing gel
    d. Shine gel
    ____

17. If a light unit has four bulbs in it, and each bulb is 9-watts, then the lamp is called a _____ lamp.
    a. 3-watt
    b. 7-watt
    c. 11-watt
    d. 36-watt
    ____

18. Different bulbs produce greatly differing amounts of UV and LED light. This is referred to as the UV and LED bulb intensity or _____.
    a. concentration
    b. strength
    c. amperage
    d. occlusion
    ____

19. After the nail pate is properly prepared for a light cured gel application, each layer of product is applied to the natural nail, nail tip, or form and requires exposure to a UV or LED light source to _____.
    a. dry
    b. cure or harden
    c. soften
    d. take polish
    ____

20. Gel polish _____.
    a. thickens over time
    b. thins out over time
    c. does not dry the same as lacquers
    d. has an odor
    ____

21. The amount of colored pigment concentration in a gel is called _____.
    a. viscosity
    b. translucence
    c. pigmentation
    d. opacity
    ____

22. Which product removes surface moisture and tiny amounts of oil left on the natural nail plate?
    a. Nail adhesive
    b. Nail dehydrator
    c. Gel primer
    d. Cleansing solution
    ____

23. If a client has flat fingernails, which type of product would be recommended?
    a. Building gel
    b. Bonding gel
    c. Self-leveling gel
    d. Glossing gel
    ____

24. During a gel procedure, keep the brush and open gel containers away from sunlight, gel lamps, and _____.
    a. terry towels
    b. metal abrasives
    c. full-spectrum table lamps
    d. manicuring implements   ____

25. Most LED lamps cure gel about four times faster than UV lamps. What do the letters *LED* represent?
    a. Light energy direction
    b. Light emitting diodes
    c. Light energy diodes
    d. Luminescent energy diodes   ____

CHAPTER 30 PREPARING FOR LICENSURE & EMPLOYMENT

1. The typical independent salon has about _____ styling stations.
   a. three
   b. five
   c. ten
   d. forty ____

2. Which type of salon shares a national name, consistent image, and business formula that is used at every location?
   a. Franchise salon
   b. Day spa
   c. Value-priced salon
   d. Medical spa ____

3. On the day of an exam, it is important to arrive early with a self-confident attitude and be alert, calm, and _____.
   a. anxious
   b. ready for a break
   c. eager to pass
   d. ready for the challenge ____

4. After doing a salon site visit, it is important to send the salon representative a _____.
   a. personal photo
   b. cover letter
   c. thank-you note
   d. resume ____

5. Which of these questions can a potential employer legally ask during an interview?
   a. How old are you?
   b. Are you authorized to work in the United States?
   c. What is your native language?
   d. What types of illnesses or disabilities do you have? ____

6. When going over the directions for the exam, if there are things you do not understand, you should _____.
   a. try to figure it out on your own
   b. turn your test in and take the exam another day
   c. focus on the parts of the exam you do understand
   d. ask the examiner ____

7. When answering a multiple choice question _____.
   a. if two choices are opposites, one is probably correct
   b. you should stop reading the choices when you see one that looks correct
   c. responses such as "all of the above" are usually not the correct choice
   d. you should never guess under any circumstances   ____

8. Which of these words is an example of an absolute?
   a. Sometimes   c. Equal
   b. Never   d. Good   ____

9. When taking the practical exam, which of the following behaviors is not likely to be beneficial?
   a. Observe other practical exams prior to taking yours if allowed to do so.
   b. Follow all infection control and safety procedures throughout the exam.
   c. Focus on what the other test candidates are doing as you work.
   d. Listen carefully to the instructions and follow them explicitly.   ____

10. Having the drive to take the necessary action to achieve a goal is known as _____.
   a. integrity   c. motivation
   b. enthusiasm   d. work ethic   ____

11. When preparing your professional resume, it is recommended that you _____.
   a. make it about two pages long
   b. focus primarily on the schools you have attended
   c. omit information about your professional skills
   d. focus on information relevant to the position you are seeking   ____

12. The process of reaching logical conclusions by employing logical reasoning is called _____.
   a. intuition   c. postulating
   b. deductive reasoning d. deciphering information   ____

13. A _____ is a written summary of a person's education and work experience.
   a. portfolio   c. cover letter
   b. personal history   d. resume   ____

14. The basic question or problem in a test question is known
as a _____.
a. stem   c. query
b. response   d. post   ____

15. Which of these terms refers to understanding the strategies
for successfully taking tests?
a. Work ethic   c. Street-smart
b. Test-wise   d. Deductive reasoning   ____

16. A(n) _____ is a collection of photos and
documents that reflect your skills, accomplishments, and
abilities in your chosen career field.
a. resume
b. cover letter
c. employment agreement
d. employment portfolio   ____

17. During your career journey, when is a great time to achieve
significant accomplishments that will strengthen your
resume?
a. After graduation
b. After obtaining your first position
c. While you are in cosmetology school
d. After achieving success   ____

18. Which of the following behaviors is not considered a good
study habit?
a. Staying up late studying the night before a test
b. Reading content carefully
c. Developing a detailed vocabulary list
d. Organizing and reviewing handouts   ____

19. Having _____ means being committed to a strong
code of moral and artistic values.
a. motivation   c. enthusiasm
b. integrity   d. a strong work ethic   ____

20. Which type of salon is most likely to offer extras such as
five-minute head, neck, and shoulder massages as part of
the shampoo?
a. High-end image salon
b. Mid-priced full-service salon
c. Booth rental salon
d. Basic value-priced salon   ____

21. When developing your resume, use concise, clear sentences and avoid overwriting or _____.
    a. direct language
    b. action verbs
    c. relevant experience
    d. flowery language ____

22. A powerful portfolio will include letters of reference from _____.
    a. friends
    b. family members
    c. former employers
    d. neighbors ____

23. It is recommend that you create a digital portfolio or _____.
    a. an online showcase of your work
    b. written summary of your career highlights
    c. limited review of accomplishments
    d. after photos of your work ____

24. Getting into the field and visiting salons and talking to salon owners, managers, educators and stylists is known as _____.
    a. visiting
    b. interacting
    c. networking
    d. speaking ____

25. What is the third step in the process of securing employment?
    a. Targeting the salon
    b. Requesting an interview
    c. Observing the salon
    d. Showing up for a spontaneous interview ____

26. Your interview outfit should be fashionable and flattering as well as similar to the salon's _____.
    a. color scheme
    b. logo colors
    c. clientele dress
    d. style culture ____

27. Important supporting materials that should be taken to an employment interview include your resume, employment portfolio, and _____.
    a. your ideas for change
    b. your medical history
    c. facts and figures
    d. your birth certificate ____

CHAPTER 31 ON THE JOB

1. It is recommended that you select which of these people as a role model?
   a. A friend
   b. A stylist in the salon
   c. A client
   d. A vendor

   ____

2. The first reality when you are in a service business is that your career revolves around _____.
   a. serving your clients
   b. making a profit
   c. making yourself happy
   d. helping your coworkers

   ____

3. Which of the following methods of compensation is not likely to be encountered in the salon industry?
   a. Salary
   b. Commission
   c. Salary plus commission
   d. Salary minus tips

   ____

4. Being a good team player includes _____.
   a. focusing on your own work
   b. withholding your knowledge
   c. refusing to be subordinate
   d. striving to help others

   ____

5. The common range for commissions is _____.
   a. 15 to 25 percent
   b. 20 to 30 percent
   c. 25 to 60 percent
   d. 50 to 80 percent

   ____

6. When is the best time to think about getting your client back into the salon?
   a. Before they arrive at the salon
   b. While they are still in the salon
   c. Just after they leave the salon
   d. Several days after they leave the salon

   ____

7. Which payment structure is often used to motivate employees to perform more services, thereby increasing their productivity?
   a. Salary plus commission
   b. Salary plus tips
   c. Hourly rate
   d. Weekly rate
   ____

8. The Internet is a powerful medium to _____ and attract new clients.
   a. share secrets
   b. build your reputation
   c. reach lost relatives
   d. improve your skills
   ____

9. The practice of recommending and selling additional services to your clients is known as _____.
   a. incentivizing
   b. retailing
   c. hard selling
   d. ticket upgrading
   ____

10. The term _____ refers to the percentage of the revenue that the salon takes in from services performed by a particular cosmetologist.
    a. salary
    b. wage
    c. commission
    d. tip
    ____

11. Which of these terms refers to customers who are loyal to a particular cosmetologist?
    a. Client base
    b. Walk-ins
    c. Loyalists
    d. Personnel
    ____

12. A(n) _____ is a document that outlines all the duties and responsibilities of a particular position in a salon or spa.
    a. employment agreement
    b. resume
    c. job description
    d. rental agreement
    ____

13. The act of recommending and selling products to your clients for at-home use is known as _____.
    a. soft selling
    b. ticketing
    c. wholesaling
    d. retailing
    ____

14. Which of these strategies will help you to effectively meet your clients' needs?
    a. Always put yourself first.
    b. Be punctual.
    c. Say whatever is necessary to make a sale.
    d. Once you have a job, stop learning and focus solely on working.
    ____

15. Which of the following information is not typically included in a job description?
  a. All of the employee's duties
  b. All of the employee's responsibilities
  c. The attitudes the employee is expected to have
  d. The specifics of the individual employee's salary ____

16. Which of these is usually the best form of compensation for a new salon professional to start out?
  a. Salary   **c.** Commission
  b. Salary plus commission   **d.** Tips ____

17. If you default, it means that you _____.
  a. opened a line of credit   **c.** failed to repay a loan
  b. were asked to leave your job   **d.** paid your bills on time ____

18. Which of these is a recommended method of increasing your income?
  a. Lowering your prices for services
  b. Spending more money
  c. Retailing less
  d. Working more hours ____

19. To become a proficient salesperson, you must be able to apply all but which of the following principles of selling salon products?
  a. Be familiar with the features and benefits of the various services and products you sell.
  b. Always use a hard sell approach, stressing why a client must purchase the product.
  c. Generate interest and desire in the customer by asking questions that determine a need.
  d. Deliver your sales talk in a relaxed, friendly manner. ____

20. There are serious consequences for not reporting cash tips as income including fines and potentially jail time as well as _____.
  a. raising your social security retirement income
  b. decreasing your borrowing power
  c. raising the Bureau of Labor's endorsement of cosmetology as a sustainable industry
  d. increasing the employer match of your 401(k) savings account ____

21. Once you understand the principles behind selling, you can also feel good about providing your clients with _____.

    a. a friendly smile   **c.** a valuable service

    b. more products than needed   **d.** a gift certificate   ____

22. A good way to get the conversation started on retailing products is to _____.

    a. place the product in the client's hands

    b. have dim, subtle lighting in the retail area

    c. rarely offer sales promotions

    d. not share the product benefits as clients will not understand them   ____

23. Make yourself available for public speaking anywhere that will put you in front of people in your community who are _____.

    a. ready to listen   **c.** potential friends

    b. potential clients   **d.** already have a stylist   ____

24. Keeping track of where your money goes is one step toward making sure that you _____.

    a. always have enough

    b. maintain confidence

    c. always have more than you need

    d. have a good work ethic   ____

25. Which of the following strategies does not represent a marketing technique that will help you expand your client base?

    a. Rush through services so that you can see more clients each day.

    b. Send clients birthday cards with special offers inside.

    c. Start a business card referral program.

    d. Be reliable, positive, and respectful of clients.   ____

32 THE SALON BUSINESS

1. When gathering accurate financial information for purchasing an existing salon, it is often helpful to consult with a(n) _____.
   a. interior designer
   b. attorney
   c. architect
   d. certified public accountant _____

2. Another name for an individual owner who determines policies and has the last say in decision making is a _____.
   a. business partner
   b. stockholder
   c. sole proprietor
   d. manager _____

3. Supplies used in the daily business operation are considered _____.
   a. retail supplies
   b. consumption supplies
   c. consumer supplies
   d. inventory supplies _____

4. Supplies purchased by a salon that are to be sold to clients are _____.
   a. retail supplies
   b. consumption supplies
   c. inventory supplies
   d. client supplies _____

5. When planning and constructing the best physical layout for a salon, the primary concern should be _____.
   a. color scheme
   b. salon furniture
   c. salon carpeting
   d. maximum efficiency _____

6. It should always be your top priority to meet which of the following financial obligations?
   a. Utility bills
   b. Vendor bills
   c. Payroll
   d. Rent or mortgage _____

7. Which of these is considered the very best form of advertising for a salon?
   a. Radio spots
   b. Satisfied clients
   c. Television ads
   d. Newspaper ads _____

8. A(n) _____ is an essential set of benchmarks that, once achieved, helps you realize your mission and your vision.
   a. assignment   **c.** obligation
   b. result   **d.** goal   ____

9. When choosing a location for your business, you should select one that _____.
   a. offers easy access   **c.** is secluded
   b. has limited parking   **d.** has low traffic   ____

10. What is the minimum number of stockholders allowed for a corporation to exist?
    a. Zero   **c.** Two
    b. One   **d.** Three   ____

11. If you operate your salon in a building that you own, it is not necessary to purchase which of the following types of insurance?
    a. Liability insurance   **c.** Renter's insurance
    b. Malpractice insurance   **d.** Burglary insurance ____

12. Which of these terms refers to your staff or employees?
    a. Personnel   **c.** Clients
    b. Constituents   **d.** Creditors   ____

13. Human resources does not cover which of the following concerns?
    a. What you can and cannot say when hiring someone
    b. What you must do when firing someone
    c. What you should do when you need to increase sales
    d. How you manage your employees   ____

14. Booking appointments is primarily whose job?
    a. The cosmetologist's   **c.** The manager's
    b. The client's   **d.** The receptionist's   ____

15. The first goal of every business should be to _____.
    a. maintain current clients
    b. attract new clients
    c. compensate employees fairly
    d. upgrade existing equipment   ____

16. Which part of a business plan outlines employees and management levels and describes how the business will be run administratively?
    a. Financial documents
    b. Organizational plan
    c. Vision statement
    d. Mission statement ____

17. Which part of a business plan summarizes your plan and states your objectives?
    a. Salon policies
    b. Marketing plan
    c. Mission statement
    d. Executive summary ____

18. Which part of a business plan includes projected financial statements, actual statements, and financial statement analyses?
    a. Organizational plan
    b. Vision statement
    c. Financial documents
    d. Salon policies ____

19. Which part of a business plan ensures that all clients and employees are treated fairly and consistently?
    a. Salon policies
    b. Financial documents
    c. Executive summary
    d. Organizational plan ____

20. Which part of a business plan is a long-term picture of what the business is to become and what it will look like when it gets there?
    a. Vision statement
    b. Mission statement
    c. Salon policies
    d. Marketing plan ____

21. Which part of a business plan outlines all of the research obtained regarding the clients your business will target and their needs, wants, and habits?
    a. Organizational plan
    b. Financial documents
    c. Marketing plan
    d. Executive summary ____

22. Which part of a business plan includes the owner's resume, personal financial information, legal contracts, and any other agreements?
    a. Executive summary
    b. Salon policies
    c. Financial documents
    d. Supporting documents ____

23. Which part of a business plan is a description of the key strategic influences of the business?
    a. Vision statement
    b. Mission statement
    c. Supporting documents
    d. Marketing plan ____

24. An agreement to buy an established salon does not typically include which of the following?
    a. An analysis of future maintenance costs
    b. A signed statement of inventory and its value
    c. A financial audit
    d. Confirmation of the identity of the owner ____

25. Costs to create even a small salon in an existing space can range from _____ per square foot.
    a. $5 to $15   c. $30 to $80
    b. $20 to $35   d. $75 to $125 ____

26. A form of business in which a firm that is already successful enters into a continuing contractual relationship with other businesses is _____.
    a. a sole proprietorship   c. a franchise
    b. a corporation   d. a partnership ____

27. Smooth business management depends on sufficient investment capital as well as _____.
    a. adequate business procedures
    b. excellent customer service delivery
    c. minimal computer skills
    d. personnel with only basic training ____

28. Someone who is trained to do everything from recording sales and payroll to generating a profit-and-loss statement is _____.
    a. a full-charge bookkeeper   c. a receptionist
    b. a financial director   d. a manager ____

29. For a cosmetologist who has a large, steady clientele and who does not have to rely on the salon's general clientele to keep busy, _____ may be a desirable situation.
    a. a franchise
    b. an S corporation
    c. a limited liability company
    d. booth rental ____

30. With each call, a gracious, appropriate response will help build _____.
    a. teamwork   c. the salon's reputation
    b. a quiet atmosphere   d. the salon's energy level ____

Note: The page numbers in italics refer to where the answer is referenced in your student textbook.

Chapter 1   HISTORY & CAREER OPPORTUNITIES

1. c, *7*	8. a, *7*	14. c, *10–11*	20. c, *10*
2. b, *7*	9. c, *8*	15. b, *12*	21. a, *17*
3. a, *7*	10. b, *9*	16. a, *12*	22. d, *11*
4. d, *9*	11. c, *9*	17. d, *16*	23. c, *12*
5. c, *9*	12. a, *9*	18. b, *17*	24. b, *11*
6. b, *8*	13. d, *11*	19. b, *17*	25. a, *11*
7. a, *8*			

Chapter 2   LIFE SKILLS

1. b, *27*	8. a, *33*	14. c, *23*	20. d, *23*
2. c, *32*	9. d, *31*	15. b, *24*	21. a, *24*
3. a, *22*	10. c, *29*	16. a, *24*	22. c, *25*
4. a, *22*	11. b, *23*	17. c, *24*	23. b, *27*
5. d, *23*	12. d, *24*	18. b, *23*	24. d, *32*
6. a, *30*	13. b, *24*	19. b, *24*	25. d, *24*
7. b, *34*			

Chapter 3   YOUR PROFESSIONAL IMAGE

1. c, *40*	8. a, *39*	14. c, *40*	20. a, *43*
2. b, *42*	9. c, *40*	15. a, *41*	21. a, *43*
3. a, *44*	10. b, *39*	16. b, *42*	22. d, *43*
4. d, *38*	11. d, *39*	17. d, *42*	23. b, *43*
5. b, *42*	12. a, *40*	18. b, *41*	24. c, *44*
6. a, *39*	13. b, *40*	19. c, *43*	25. b, *41*
7. c, *42*			

Chapter 4   COMMUNICATING FOR SUCCESS

1. c, *48*	8. d, *56*	14. b, *63*	20. b, *51*
2. b, *60*	9. a, *59*	15. c, *63*	21. c, *56*
3. d, *48*	10. d, *61*	16. b, *50*	22. b, *59*
4. c, *56*	11. c, *62*	17. a, *50*	23. b, *60*
5. b, *49*	12. b, *62*	18. c, *54*	24. a, *50*
6. a, *49*	13. a, *61*	19. a, *54*	25. b, *58*
7. c, *50*			

Chapter 5   INFECTION CONTROL: PRINCIPLES & PRACTICES

1. a, *77*	4. c, *77*	7. a, *78*	10. c, *84*
2. d, *77*	5. a, *76*	8. c, *79*	11. a, *84*
3. a, *77*	6. c, *78*	9. b, *79*	12. d, *74, 86*

13. c, *93*   29. b, *83*   45. b, *104*   61. d, *80*
14. c, *71*   30. d, *89*   46. b, *81*   62. d, *81*
15. d, *88*   31. d, *84*   47. d, *76*   63. c, *83*
16. b, *104*   32. c, *86*   48. d, *78*   64. c, *78*
17. b, *93*   33. a, *88*   49. c, *78*   65. b, *81*
18. a, *93*   34. d, *88*   50. b, *78*   66. d, *83*
19. d, *72*   35. b, *88*   51. a, *80*   67. a, *81*
20. b, *100*   36. b, *88*   52. b, *75*   68. c, *81*
21. a, *100*   37. d, *110*   53. b, *72*   69. b, *81*
22. b, *82*   38. c, *90*   54. d, *76*   70. a, *72*
23. d, *87*   39. b, *92*   55. c, *85*   71. d, *75*
24. b, *97*   40. a, *73*   56. a, *81*   72. b, *77*
25. b, *71*   41. b, *93*   57. d, *81*   73. c, *81*
26. d, *74*   42. c, *94*   58. b, *81*   74. b, *86*
27. b, *72*   43. d, *96*   59. c, *81*   75. a, *89*
28. c, *82*   44. a, *103*   60. b, *80*

Chapter 6   GENERAL ANATOMY & PHYSIOLOGY

1. b, *115*   15. d, *122*   29. a, *125*   43. d, *143*
2. c, *116*   16. a, *120*   30. c, *131*   44. b, *132*
3. b, *116*   17. c, *122*   31. b, *132*   45. d, *118*
4. c, *116*   18. b, *123*   32. c, *129*   46. a, *138*
5. a, *115*   19. a, *126*   33. a, *132*   47. d, *137*
6. d, *117*   20. d, *126*   34. d, *131*   48. b, *122*
7. b, *117*   21. d, *128*   35. b, *134*   49. d, *128*
8. d, *117*   22. b, *129*   36. c, *134*   50. a, *140*
9. b, *119*   23. c, *133*   37. b, *135*   51. c, *118*
10. c, *121*   24. b, *136*   38. a, *138*   52. a, *118*
11. a, *143*   25. a, *136*   39. d, *139*   53. d, *115*
12. b, *120*   26. b, *124*   40. c, *130*   54. d, *128*
13. a, *119*   27. c, *125*   41. b, *132*   55. b, *137*
14. b, *121*   28. d, *130*   42. a, *137*

Chapter 7   SKIN STRUCTURE, GROWTH, & NUTRITION

1. b, *154*   10. b, *158*   19. b, *164*   28. a, *160*
2. a, *155*   11. a, *159*   20. a, *162*   29. b, *161*
3. a, *155*   12. d, *159*   21. c, *163*   30. c, *157*
4. d, *156–157*   13. d, *160–161*   22. c, *164*   31. b, *161*
5. a, *156*   14. d, *163*   23. b, *165*   32. a, *156*
6. c, *157*   15. b, *165*   24. d, *165*   33. d, *156*
7. a, *157*   16. c, *156*   25. a, *162*   34. a, *161*
8. d, *158*   17. d, *155*   26. c, *157*   35. d, *156*
9. c, *158*   18. a, *162*   27. d, *156*

Chapter 8 SKIN DISORDERS & DISEASES

1. d, *186*	10. b, *182*	19. c, *187*	28. b, *176*
2. c, *188*	11. c, *173*	20. b, *190*	29. c, *175*
3. a, *174*	12. d, *178*	21. d, *175*	30. d, *174*
4. d, *176*	13. c, *180*	22. b, *178*	31. b, *183*
5. a, *178*	14. a, *181*	23. a, *174*	32. a, *184*
6. c, *177*	15. b, *178*	24. d, *179*	33. c, *187*
7. a, *179*	16. d, *184*	25. b, *177*	34. b, *189*
8. b, *180*	17. c, *185*	26. a, *179*	35. b, *179*
9. d, *180*	18. b, *185*	27. a, *175*	

Chapter 9 NAIL STRUCTURE & GROWTH

1. c, *198*	8. b, *203*	14. b, *200*	20. c, *203*
2. a, *199*	9. a, *202*	15. d, *201*	21. a, *200*
3. b, *200*	10. d, *198*	16. c, *201*	22. b, *199*
4. a, *199*	11. c, *198*	17. c, *200*	23. d, *201*
5. b, *201*	12. a, *198*	18. b, *202*	24. d, *200*
6. d, *201*	13. c, *199*	19. c, *203*	25. c, *200*
7. c, *200*			

Chapter 10 NAIL DISORDERS & DISEASES

1. a, *208*	9. b, *212*	17. c, *214*	25. d, *212*
2. b, *211*	10. c, *215*	18. a, *213*	26. a, *214*
3. b, *216*	11. a, *218*	19. d, *212–213*	27. b, *214*
4. d, *216*	12. b, *214*	20. c, *213*	28. c, *214*
5. c, *214*	13. d, *210*	21. b, *209*	29. b, *218*
6. b, *211*	14. c, *209*	22. b, *210*	30. a, *218*
7. c, *214*	15. b, *209*	23. a, *210*	
8. c, *208–209*	16. a, *210*	24. c, *211*	

Chapter 11 PROPERTIES OF THE HAIR & SCALP

1. b, *224*	14. c, *232*	27. c, *228*	40. c, *227*
2. c, *224*	15. b, *242*	28. d, *233*	41. d, *240*
3. a, *225*	16. a, *244*	29. b, *233*	42. c, *241*
4. c, *225*	17. d, *244*	30. d, *233*	43. b, *242*
5. b, *225*	18. c, *245*	31. c, *233*	44. d, *243*
6. d, *225*	19. b, *247*	32. a, *234*	45. d, *243*
7. c, *226*	20. d, *232*	33. d, *234*	46. a, *226*
8. b, *227*	21. d, *233*	34. d, *235*	47. c, *225*
9. a, *232*	22. c, *232–233*	35. c, *235*	48. a, *228*
10. d, *227*	23. a, *237*	36. a, *236*	49. d, *227*
11. b, *228*	24. c, *238*	37. a, *237*	50. c, *236*
12. a, *230*	25. b, *239*	38. b, *239*	51. b, *238*
13. a, *230*	26. a, *225*	39. d, *239*	52. c, *239*

53. b, *225*   58. c, *240*   63. d, *246*   68. b, *235*
54. a, *238*   59. b, *224*   64. a, *224*   69. a, *232*
55. b, *241*   60. d, *232*   65. d, *247*   70. a, *240*
56. c, *228*   61. a, *238*   66. b, *244*
57. d, *233*   62. c, *227*   67. a, *227*

Chapter 12   BASICS OF CHEMISTRY

1. c, *255*   10. c, *262*   19. c, *259*   28. c, *255*
2. d, *255*   11. d, *265*   20. b, *259*   29. a, *258*
3. b, *256*   12. a, *266*   21. d, *261*   30. d, *259*
4. a, *260*   13. b, *259*   22. a, *263*   31. c, *259*
5. c, *260*   14. c, *266*   23. b, *264*   32. b, *269*
6. d, *261*   15. a, *264*   24. a, *264*   33. d, *259*
7. a, *261*   16. d, *255*   25. b, *258*   34. d, *257*
8. b, *261*   17. a, *256*   26. b, *265*
9. b, *262*   18. c, *257*   27. a, *258*

Chapter 13   BASICS OF ELECTRICITY

1. b, *274*   9. d, *280*   17. d, *285*   25. d, *287*
2. a, *275*   10. b, *281*   18. d, *285*   26. a, *279*
3. c, *275*   11. b, *278*   19. a, *286*   27. c, *282*
4. b, *275*   12. b, *279*   20. c, *286*   28. b, *285*
5. d, *276*   13. d, *280*   21. a, *280*   29. d, *287*
6. a, *277*   14. b, *281*   22. b, *281*   30. c, *277*
7. a, *278*   15. c, *283*   23. c, *288*
8. c, *278*   16. b, *284*   24. d, *282*

Chapter 14   PRINCIPLES OF HAIR DESIGN

1. b, *300*   10. b, *316*   19. d, *314*   28. a, *310*
2. c, *302*   11. a, *300*   20. d, *317*   29. b, *312*
3. a, *303*   12. c, *306*   21. a, *298*   30. c, *317*
4. b, *303*   13. c, *306*   22. b, *298*   31. d, *309*
5. d, *304*   14. a, *307*   23. a, *298*   32. b, *302*
6. a, *304*   15. d, *308*   24. d, *299*   33. a, *301*
7. c, *304*   16. a, *313*   25. c, *299*   34. c, *296–297*
8. d, *310*   17. a, *314*   26. d, *310*   35. c, *311*
9. d, *312*   18. b, *315*   27. b, *311*

Chapter 15   SCALP CARE, SHAMPOOING, & CONDITIONING

1. b, *327*   6. c, *335*   11. b, *349*   16. d, *324*
2. d, *329*   7. d, *336*   12. d, *325*   17. a, *328*
3. a, *330*   8. b, *336*   13. b, *323*   18. d, *334*
4. a, *330*   9. a, *326*   14. c, *325*   19. b, *335*
5. b, *332*   10. c, *326*   15. a, *349*   20. d, *336*

21. a, *336*	26. a, *330*	31. a, *332*	36. b, *335*
22. d, *336*	27. b, *330*	32. a, *333*	37. a, *333*
23. c, *339*	28. d, *324*	33. c, *333*	38. c, *329*
24. a, *340*	29. c, *332*	34. c, *330*	39. b, *327*
25. b, *343*	30. b, *332*	35. d, *337*	40. d, *330*

Chapter 16 HAIRCUTTING

1. c, *360*	20. d, *393*	39. c, *372*	58. b, *362*
2. b, *362*	21. c, *394*	40. a, *373*	59. a, *361*
3. c, *362*	22. a, *396*	41. d, *376*	60. d, *362*
4. d, *362*	23. d, *396*	42. d, *378*	61. d, *362*
5. c, *363*	24. b, *401*	43. a, *378*	62. a, *362*
6. a, *364–365*	25. a, *373*	44. d, *380*	63. b, *387*
7. b, *366*	26. c, *358*	45. b, *387*	64. c, *374*
8. b, *367*	27. a, *363*	46. b, *370, 392*	65. d, *375*
9. d, *363*	28. d, *364*	47. d, *394*	66. b, *376*
10. d, *368*	29. b, *373*	48. b, *401*	67. a, *377*
11. b, *371*	30. b, *380*	49. c, *403*	68. c, *381*
12. c, *379*	31. d, *389*	50. a, *358*	69. b, *383*
13. a, *380*	32. a, *366*	51. c, *359*	70. d, *384*
14. b, *381*	33. d, *367*	52. b, *359*	71. c, *388*
15. d, *381*	34. c, *367*	53. c, *359*	72. a, *389*
16. b, *382*	35. b, *368*	54. a, *359*	73. c, *394*
17. a, *384*	36. d, *368*	55. d, *360*	74. d, *400*
18. c, *385*	37. d, *370*	56. b, *361*	75. b, *363*
19. b, *390*	38. a, *371*	57. a, *361*	

Chapter 17 HAIRSTYLING

1. c, *444*	18. a, *467*	34. b, *465*	50. b, *457*
2. b, *445*	19. b, *469*	35. a, *468*	51. d, *458*
3. d, *446*	20. b, *473*	36. a, *468*	52. a, *458*
4. a, *446*	21. c, *461*	37. a, *469*	53. a, *444*
5. d, *447*	22. a, *451*	38. b, *448*	54. c, *448*
6. a, *447*	23. c, *452*	39. c, *448*	55. b, *451*
7. b, *448*	24. d, *473*	40. d, *448*	56. a, *451*
8. c, *449*	25. a, *453*	41. a, *449*	57. b, *453*
9. c, *451*	26. d, *456*	42. d, *449*	58. d, *447*
10. d, *451*	27. b, *456*	43. b, *450*	59. c, *457*
11. a, *452*	28. d, *457*	44. c, *450*	60. a, *459*
12. b, *454*	29. c, *460*	45. a, *452*	61. b, *465*
13. d, *458*	30. d, *461*	46. b, *452*	62. d, *470*
14. c, *459*	31. a, *462*	47. d, *454*	63. c, *471*
15. b, *459*	32. c, *463*	48. c, *454*	64. a, *472*
16. c, *462*	33. b, *465*	49. c, *457*	65. b, *473*
17. a, *467*			

Chapter 18 BRAIDING & BRAID EXTENSIONS

1. c, *528*	11. a, *528*	21. b, *542*	31. c, *534*
2. d, *539*	12. b, *532*	22. d, *532*	32. d, *536*
3. b, *539*	13. b, *533*	23. a, *531*	33. a, *538*
4. b, *531*	14. c, *535*	24. c, *532*	34. d, *532*
5. a, *533–534*	15. c, *536*	25. a, *538*	35. b, *533*
6. d, *534*	16. b, *540*	26. b, *532*	36. c, *529*
7. c, *535*	17. a, *542*	27. d, *532*	37. a, *530*
8. a, *537*	18. b, *542*	28. c, *532*	38. b, *539*
9. b, *537*	19. d, *542*	29. b, *537*	39. d, *540*
10. d, *543*	20. c, *536*	30. a, *532*	40. c, *541*

Chapter 19 WIGS & HAIR ADDITIONS

1. a, *573*	10. d, *591*	19. d, *577*	28. b, *574*
2. c, *575*	11. b, *574*	20. b, *584*	29. d, *576*
3. d, *580*	12. a, *581*	21. c, *579*	30. a, *579*
4. b, *580*	13. c, *581*	22. a, *586*	31. d, *588*
5. c, *578*	14. b, *585*	23. c, *578*	32. b, *585*
6. a, *582*	15. d, *588*	24. d, *576*	33. c, *582*
7. b, *582*	16. b, *590*	25. a, *577*	34. a, *582*
8. a, *588*	17. b, *592*	26. b, *577*	35. a, *581*
9. d, *589*	18. a, *584*	27. c, *576*	

Chapter 20 CHEMICAL TEXTURE SERVICES

1. b, *598*	18. a, *610*	34. b, *603*	50. c, *613*
2. c, *599*	19. d, *611*	35. c, *599*	51. b, *667*
3. b, *599*	20. a, *604*	36. d, *614*	52. d, *600*
4. d, *602*	21. b, *599*	37. b, *600*	53. a, *619*
5. a, *612*	22. a, *602*	38. a, *612*	54. c, *601*
6. b, *612*	23. c, *603*	39. b, *618*	55. b, *603*
7. a, *602*	24. d, *604*	40. d, *621*	56. d, *603*
8. a, *604*	25. b, *604*	41. c, *599*	57. b, *604*
9. c, *604*	26. d, *605*	42. b, *612*	58. a, *604*
10. b, *605*	27. a, *606*	43. d, *611*	59. d, *604*
11. d, *608*	28. c, *616*	44. a, *614*	60. c, *605*
12. a, *617*	29. b, *618*	45. c, *617*	61. a, *606*
13. b, *618*	30. a, *618*	46. a, *610*	62. b, *608*
14. a, *622*	31. d, *620*	47. b, *618*	63. c, *608*
15. c, *620*	32. a, *610*	48. a, *599*	64. d, *618*
16. b, *620*	33. c, *610*	49. d, *611*	65. b, *622*
17. c, *601*			

Chapter 21 HAIRCOLORING

1. a, 672
2. c, 672
3. d, 672
4. b, 673
5. b, 678
6. a, 678
7. d, 678
8. c, 676
9. d, 676
10. a, 676
11. b, 676
12. c, 676
13. d, 677
14. d, 680
15. b, 680
16. a, 681
17. b, 681
18. d, 684
19. c, 685
20. b, 694
21. a, 695
22. d, 699
23. a, 702
24. b, 702
25. c, 704
26. a, 696
27. c, 706
28. d, 707
29. c, 678
30. a, 678
31. b, 679
32. d, 681
33. b, 686
34. c, 685
35. a, 691
36. b, 693
37. d, 697
38. b, 678
39. d, 684
40. c, 673
41. a, 695
42. d, 682
43. b, 685
44. a, 698
45. d, 673
46. b, 691
47. c, 684
48. b, 683
49. d, 682
50. c, 693
51. c, 672
52. a, 705–706
53. a, 683
54. c, 706
55. d, 699
56. b, 675
57. a, 693
58. d, 673
59. c, 695
60. b, 683
61. a, 692
62. d, 674
63. a, 676
64. b, 679
65. c, 680
66. b, 682
67. b, 683
68. d, 689
69. c, 692
70. c, 699
71. a, 700
72. c, 701
73. b, 705
74. d, 706
75. a, 694

Chapter 22 HAIR REMOVAL

1. c, 739
2. b, 744
3. b, 744
4. a, 745
5. c, 746
6. a, 747
7. d, 747
8. a, 747
9. d, 756
10. c, 760
11. a, 746
12. b, 744
13. c, 746
14. d, 745
15. b, 743
16. a, 742–743
17. b, 738
18. d, 746
19. c, 746
20. a, 746
21. b, 746
22. d, 744
23. a, 738
24. c, 743
25. d, 744

Chapter 23 FACIALS

1. a, 772
2. b, 772
3. a, 773
4. d, 773
5. c, 773
6. b, 773
7. d, 774
8. a, 774
9. c, 775
10. a, 776
11. d, 778
12. c, 780
13. d, 781
14. a, 782
15. c, 782
16. b, 783
17. b, 788
18. c, 789
19. a, 790
20. d, 795
21. a, 768
22. c, 774
23. b, 777
24. d, 778
25. c, 778
26. b, 779
27. a, 779
28. a, 777
29. d, 773
30. b, 779
31. c, 773
32. b, 775
33. a, 789
34. c, 773
35. d, 777
36. a, 778
37. b, 782
38. c, 776
39. b, 780
40. d, 767
41. c, 776
42. a, 774
43. d, 768
44. b, 772
45. d, 774
46. a, 778
47. b, 779
48. c, 781
49. b, 782
50. d, 782

Chapter 24 FACIAL MAKEUP

1. b, *813*	10. a, *827*	19. a, *812*	28. a, *816*
2. b, *818*	11. d, *820*	20. b, *816*	29. c, *817*
3. d, *823*	12. b, *823*	21. d, *815*	30. b, *834*
4. c, *818*	13. d, *823*	22. c, *815*	31. a, *816*
5. a, *828, 830*	14. c, *826*	23. a, *813*	32. d, *821*
6. c, *821*	15. a, *827*	24. b, *814*	33. c, *822*
7. d, *832*	16. c, *814*	25. b, *815*	34. b, *824*
8. c, *824*	17. b, *814*	26. c, *813*	35. c, *828*
9. b, *825*	18. d, *816*	27. d, *831*	

Chapter 25 MANICURING

1. b, *852*	10. b, *853*	19. b, *854*	28. d, *872*
2. a, *860*	11. d, *856*	20. c, *873*	29. a, *853*
3. b, *864*	12. a, *861*	21. a, *856*	30. d, *858*
4. c, *861*	13. d, *861*	22. d, *866*	31. c, *865*
5. d, *863*	14. c, *862*	23. b, *872*	32. b, *869*
6. c, *869*	15. b, *862*	24. a, *860*	33. b, *869*
7. a, *851*	16. c, *863*	25. c, *857*	34. a, *869*
8. c, *859*	17. c, *864*	26. d, *872*	35. c, *875*
9. d, *852*	18. d, *872*	27. b, *857*	

Chapter 26 PEDICURING

1. c, *915*	8. b, *908*	14. b, *912*	20. a, *905*
2. b, *904*	9. c, *911*	15. d, *914*	21. a, *908*
3. c, *908*	10. a, *915*	16. a, *906*	22. c, *910–911*
4. a, *914*	11. a, *904*	17. c, *906*	23. d, *911*
5. d, *916*	12. c, *909*	18. b, *905*	24. c, *912*
6. b, *901*	13. d, *911–912*	19. c, *913*	25. d, *916*
7. a, *903–904*			

Chapter 27 NAIL TIPS & WRAPS

1. b, *928*	8. b, *934*	14. d, *932*	20. a, *934*
2. a, *929*	9. d, *940*	15. c, *932*	21. d, *929*
3. b, *930*	10. b, *929*	16. b, *932*	22. c, *929*
4. d, *931*	11. a, *932*	17. d, *930*	23. b, *934*
5. d, *932*	12. c, *930*	18. b, *933*	24. a, *934*
6. c, *932*	13. a, *932*	19. c, *933*	25. d, *929–930*
7. d, *929*			

Chapter 28 MONOMER LIQUID & POLYMER POWDER NAIL ENHANCEMENTS

1. b, *952*
2. b, *953*
3. a, *955*
4. c, *960*
5. d, *961*
6. c, *969*
7. d, *957*
8. b, *958*
9. c, *961*

10. a, *963*
11. a, *961*
12. c, *962*
13. b, *954*
14. d, *953*
15. b, *952*
16. d, *952*
17. a, *954*
18. b, *956*

19. d, *956*
20. a, *956*
21. c, *959*
22. a, *963*
23. b, *963*
24. d, *954*
25. c, *955*
26. c, *959*
27. a, *960*

28. c, *963*
29. b, *963*
30. a, *964*
31. d, *958*
32. c, *966*
33. b, *966*

Chapter 29 LIGHT CURED GELS

1. c, *988–989*
2. b, *998*
3. d, *998*
4. a, *992*
5. c, *1004*
6. b, *990*
7. c, *991*

8. d, *991*
9. a, *991*
10. d, *989*
11. b, *992*
12. a, *1001*
13. d, *1001*

14. c, *989*
15. c, *992*
16. b, *992*
17. d, *997*
18. a, *998*
19. b, *989–990*

20. c, *992*
21. d, *993*
22. b, *994*
23. a, *996*
24. c, *995, 998*
25. b, *997*

Chapter 30 PREPARING FOR LICENSURE & EMPLOYMENT

1. b, *1033*
2. a, *1035*
3. d, *1028*
4. c, *1044*
5. b, *1051*
6. d, *1028*
7. a, *1030*

8. b, *1029*
9. c, *1030–1031*
10. c, *1033*
11. d, *1006*
12. b, *1029*
13. d, *1036*
14. a, *1029*

15. b, *1027*
16. d, *1040*
17. c, *1037*
18. a, *1027*
19. b, *1033*
20. a, *1035*
21. d, *1038*

22. c, *1040*
23. a, *1041*
24. c, *1043*
25. b, *1045*
26. d, *1047*
27. c, *1048*

Chapter 31 ON THE JOB

1. b, *1062*
2. a, *1058*
3. d, *1060*
4. d, *1059*
5. c, *1061*
6. b, *1073*
7. a, *1061*

8. b, *1073*
9. d, *1067*
10. c, *1061*
11. a, *1065, 1067*
12. c, *1060*
13. d, *1067*

14. b, *1058*
15. d, *1060*
16. a, *1061*
17. c, *1064*
18. d, *1065, 1067*
19. b, *1069–1070*

20. b, *1064*
21. c, *1069*
22. a, *1071*
23. b, *1073*
24. a, *1065*
25. a, *1072*

Chapter 32 THE SALON BUSINESS

1. d, *1081*
2. c, *1082*
3. b, *1088*
4. a, *1088*
5. d, *1090*
6. c, *1093*
7. b, *1097*
8. d, *1080*
9. a, *1081*
10. b, *1083*
11. c, *1086*
12. a, *1091*
13. c, *1093*
14. d, *1094*
15. a, *1099*
16. b, *1084*
17. d, *1084*
18. c, *1084*
19. a, *1084*
20. a, *1084*
21. c, *1084*
22. d, *1084*
23. b, *1084*
24. a, *1085*
25. d, *1091*
26. c, *1083*
27. b, *1087*
28. a, *1087*
29. d, *1089*
30. c, *1095*

NOTES